# Plant–Based
# INTERMITTENT
# FASTING

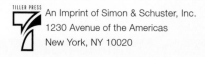 An Imprint of Simon & Schuster, Inc.
1230 Avenue of the Americas
New York, NY 10020

Conceived and produced by Elwin Street Productions Limited
14 Clerkenwell Green
London EC1R 0DP

This publication contains the opinions and ideas of its author. It is intended to provide helpful and informative material on the subjects addressed in the publication. It is sold with the understanding that the author and publisher are not engaged in rendering medical, health, or any other kind of personal, professional services in the book. The reader should consult his or her medical, health, or other competent professional before adopting any of the suggestions in this book or drawing inferences from it.

The author and publisher specifically disclaim all responsibility for any liability, loss, or risk, personal or otherwise, that is incurred as a consequence, directly or indirectly, of the use and application of any of the contents of this book.

First Tiller Press trade paperback edition in North America May 2020

TILLER PRESS and colophon are trademarks of Simon & Schuster, Inc.

For information about special discounts for bulk purchases, please contact Simon & Schuster Special Sales at 1-866-506-1949 or business@simonandschuster.com.

The Simon & Schuster Speakers Bureau can bring authors to your live event. For more information or to book an event, contact the Simon & Schuster Speakers Bureau at 1-866-248-3049 or visit our website at www.simonspeakers.com.

Photo Credits
Alamy: pp. 79, 92, 121, 141; Libby Limon: pp. 72, 105, 135, 137; Getty: p.10; Shutterstock: pp. 6, 16, 22, 32, 50, 75, 81, 85, 89, 95, 99, 103, 106, 111, 115, 117, 118, 127, 131, 139

Manufactured in Singapore

10 9 8 7 6 5 4 3 2 1

Library of Congress Cataloging-in-Publication Data has been applied for.

ISBN 978-1-9821-5093-8

# Plant–Based INTERMITTENT FASTING

## RECIPES AND MEAL PLANS FOR SUSTAINED WEIGHT LOSS, A HEALTHY METABOLISM, AND CLARITY OF MIND

## LIBBY LIMON

TILLER PRESS

New York  London  Toronto  Sydney  New Delhi

# CONTENTS

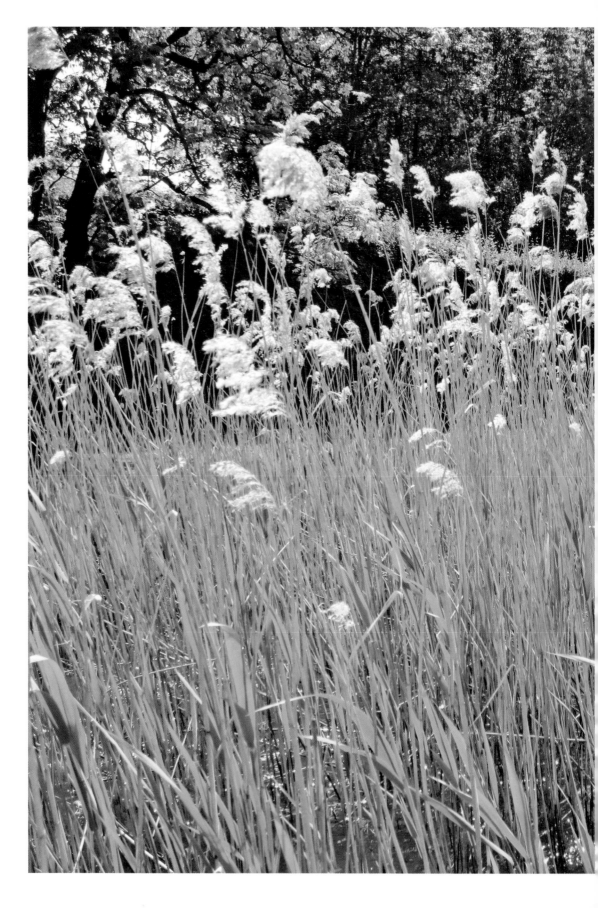

# INTRODUCTION

Over the last few decades, nutritional science has undergone a transformation, moving on from the basic knowledge of how we can prevent malnutrition to how we can use nutrition to enhance our well-being and longevity and prevent illness. Research studies into every kind of diet imaginable have been conducted, many with conflicting outcomes. However, there are a few areas that have emerged as revolutionary strategies with the potential to transform our health. Intermittent fasting, also known as "time-restricted eating," and the movement toward a plant-based diet with an increased emphasis on vegetarian and vegan foods are two of these standout examples. This book is designed to help you start integrating them into your daily life.

## The eco impact

Intermittent fasting and a plant-based diet also have potential benefits for the sustainability of the planet. In most of our planet's long history, humans have lived without hugely impacting our environment and have struggled for survival with the rest of life on earth. However, our way of living has transformed over the last few hundred years, our population has exploded, and we have arrived at an age when our standard of living and life expectancy have never been better. On the flip side, we're suffering from overconsumption, both as individuals and of the planet's resources.

## A plant-based diet

A plant-based diet includes the obvious fruits and vegetables, but just as important are other plant-based foods, such as nuts and seeds, legumes, plant-based fats and oils, herbs and spices, and even teas and coffees. Including more plant-based foods in your diet is beneficial for everyone, regardless of whether you're a dedicated vegan or a committed omnivore. A 2017 study found that reducing animal products in the diet by just 3 percent can have a significant positive effect on health, and while many will argue that we're designed to be omnivores, this shouldn't mean a meat-heavy diet. The balance in the Western diet has become distorted, and bringing your food intake back to a place where plants are of equal importance is a great way to optimize your health.

## INTERMITTENT FASTING (IF)

IF has come to prominence over the last five years. Initially the most popular strategy was the 5:2 format, which involved five days of "normal" eating, with an average intake of 2000 calories for adults, and two (usually nonconsecutive) days of fasting at 500 calories. However, many people felt that the fast days were quite taxing, encroaching on social life and work commitments. Basically, it felt like hard work, and any strategy that feels like work or as though you're missing out in some way will be a struggle to sustain.

Further research into different fasting and eating windows brought to light another strategy, known as 16:8. This requires fasting for sixteen hours and eating in an eight-hour window, which for most of us is fairly simple to slot into existing work, family, socializing, and exercising schedules. This is a plan that can work long term, resulting in improvements in energy, focus, cellular health, anti-aging efforts, anti-inflammatory efforts, and weight and body composition management.

### The fourteen-day plans

This book will guide you through two practical fourteen-day plans using the 16:8 fasting protocol. One plan is aimed at optimal health, the other at kick-starting weight loss. Their aim is to inspire, educate, and make it easy for you to begin a journey that you can continue. The plan will help you get started with two weeks of wholly plant-based recipes that will introduce vegan cooking ideas. After the two weeks, the plan can be maintained or combined with dishes from your own repertoire. These nutrition strategies can be used consistently or periodically for a well-being reset whenever you feel the need.

# ABOUT THIS BOOK

Starting a journey to detox or change our eating patterns requires more than just knowing the technical details. While knowledge about nutrition and what's good for our body is essential, integrating it into everyday life can be tricky; our eating habits are determined by personal likes and dislikes, as well as by our work and social life.

The plant-based intermittent fasting diet plans in this book are designed to fit in with your lifestyle, whether your aim is improving overall health or losing weight. They help you design your own fasting and eating windows—taking into account what suits your lifestyle and needs and introducing you to the best way to ease into each plan—achieve better and long-lasting results, and integrate exercise into your new routine.

The introductory section guides you through the benefits of intermittent fasting techniques and a plant-based diet. The diet is suitable for longtime vegans as well as non-vegans who simply want to enjoy the benefits of a plant-based detox for a limited period. The pantry section (pages 23–25) is especially useful if you aren't familiar with a plant-based diet, guiding you through the best way to organize your shopping and stock the ideal ingredients to support the plans. Any other questions you may have will be covered in the All You Need to Know section (page 32).

The two meal plans that follow are tailored to the specific goals of achieving optimal health or weight loss. The first plan is perfect if you need an energy boost while maintaining your weight, and the second one helps you start a balanced and healthy weight-loss journey.

Finally, the recipe section contains forty-five recipes, from breakfast options to mini meals, soups, salads, and main dishes, all of them nutritious and guaranteed to make your journey both delicious and effective.

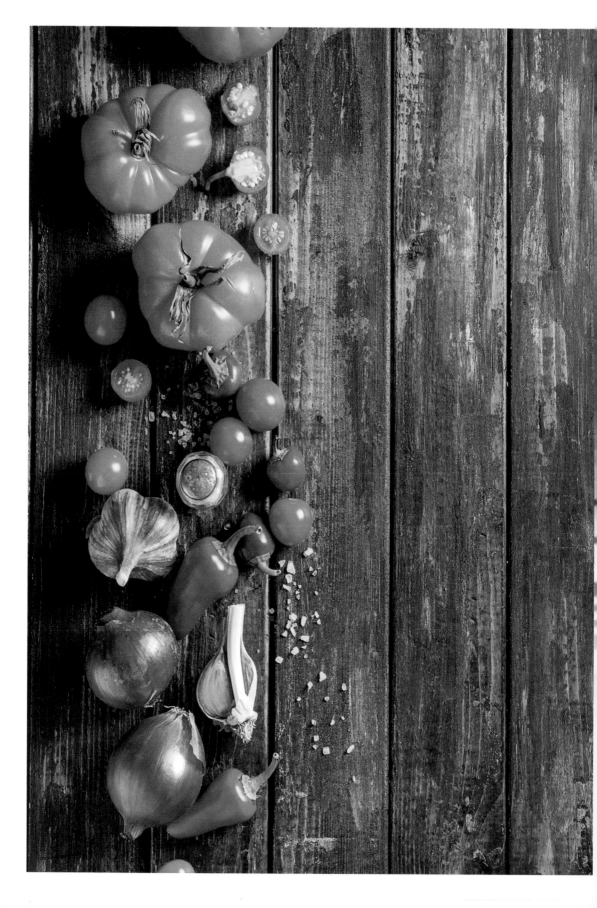

# INTERMITTENT FASTING
## —The Why and the How

So why does intermittent fasting work so well for us? The predominant theory is that the majority of human evolution took place while we were hunter-gatherers. During this period, food was not necessarily readily available, so involuntary intermittent fasts were common. Equally, it may have been necessary to hunt or gather on an empty stomach in a fasting state, and we therefore evolved to function efficiently on an empty stomach in order to survive and continue to feed ourselves.

Some historians are cautious about these theories, pointing out that with small and nomadic communities, food probably wasn't as scarce as we may think. Also, the life expectancy of humans back then was much lower than it is now, so they didn't have the same length of time to develop many of the health issues that come with age, and it is therefore difficult to gauge the extent to which their diets were linked to developing a healthy biochemistry.

Another area that directly relates to how we have evolved and how that can affect our health and well-being involves our circadian rhythm. This is our internal body clock, which tells us to be awake and eat during the day and to fast and rest at night. Working against this light-dark cycle can have a negative effect on our health, contributing to aging, weight gain, and development of disease. And it isn't just sleep that affects our circadian rhythm but also when we eat.

### The benefits of intermittent fasting

While there is debate over the origins of IF, the theory of hormesis is the overriding explanation of why it works. Hormesis is the process by which a small amount of an environmental trigger produces a small stress effect on the body that in turn causes an adaptation to improve health and well-being, making the body's systems more effective and robust. However, if that same trigger occurred in a larger amount, it would actually have a negative effect on the body. An example of this is exercise: doing the right amount makes you stronger and fitter, but overexercising leads to stress, injury, and illness.

From a food perspective, phytochemicals found in some plants are hormetins. Many of these have previously been labeled antioxidants, such as epigallocatechin gallate (EGCG) in green tea, resveratrol in red wine, and curcumin in turmeric, but they actually work by stimulating a minor stress response in the body's organs. In large amounts, however, they would have a toxic effect.

Intermittent fasting plays a key role in creating a hormetic effect on the body. If we fast for a short period, it forces the body to become more efficient and use its internal resources. However, fasting for too long can be detrimental, in some cases leading to the adaptation of "starvation" mode. When integrating IF into your life, it's important to understand this principle. We are all biochemically individual—we all have different "sweet spots" at which we achieve optimal hormesis—so some people will be able to fast for longer than others. In addition, the length of your optimal fast may change throughout your life in relation to other biochemical or environmental factors, such as infections, pregnancy, exercise regime, and nutritional status.

### Improved function, energy, and focus

Fatigue is now commonplace in our society. So many of us lack vitality and feel everyday exhaustion, fueled by busy, stressful lives, poor diet, and poor sleep, and it's in the mitochondria—the powerhouses of the cells—that this poor energy production starts. Hormesis strategies such as IF have the ability to revitalize the quality of our mitochondria, and therefore our energy levels.

Hundreds and thousands of mitochondria exist in every one of our cells. They're responsible, with the help of oxygen, for turning the nutritional resources that we give our bodies into energy we can use. Everything we do requires energy, so making sure our mitochondria are as fit as they can be has a huge impact on our well-being.

Mitochondria work by burning either glucose or fats to make the energy molecule adenosine triphosphate (ATP), which is used to power cells in everything from your brain to your immune system. Mitochondria will, as a preference, burn glucose if it's available, either from the food you eat or from glycogen stores in the liver or muscles. However, when there isn't any glucose available, they will switch to burning fats to produce ketones to drive the production of ATP. This switch—known as intermittent metabolic switching (IMS)—can be hugely beneficial to health and well-being, enhancing the number and quality of the mitochondria we have and promoting the recognition of cells that either need to be repaired, or destroyed if they are no longer useful or healthy. IF is designed to help the body make this shift to burning stored fats or ketones.

## INFLAMMATION: A MODERN-DAY EPIDEMIC

IF has the potential to reduce chronic inflammation. Inflammation can be visualized easily as a red, sore, and angry wound, or inflamed tonsils, and is an important part of an immune response to injury or infection. However, what we're understanding more and more is that chronic inflammation—an imbalanced immune response—is a major driver in the development of diseases such as heart disease, dementia, and cancer. These are often perceived as things that happen "to" us, but unlike infectious disease, they're actually things that are happening "in" us, which allows us to gain influence over them and take control of our current and future health.

Signs of chronic inflammation are the same as those associated with the stresses of modern life. Long-lasting inflammation is one of the biological causes of aches and pains, fatigue, poor sleep, functional gut issues, seasonal allergies, weight gain, and frequent low-grade illness. Excess adipose (fat) tissue also drives pro-inflammatory biological messengers.

IF has been shown to help reduce inflammatory markers, indicating it as a simple antidote. It also has the potential to improve body composition and drive fat-burning from the body's stores. This in turn will have a positive effect on the levels of inflammation in the body.

---

*One of the reasons people are resistant to integrating fasting into their daily lives is the apprehension that it will leave them tired or without the focus needed to complete daily work tasks. Actually, the opposite is likely to occur. The brain and neurological cells thrive on ketones, and regular IF can improve both their structure and function, thus improving daily productivity, mood, and long-term brain health. IF is also a healthy method of losing weight, leaving you more energized and highly focused.*

# IF AND WEIGHT MANAGEMENT

Obesity is one of the biggest health epidemics of the modern age, with around 50 percent of the population of developed nations being clinically obese. We are increasingly obsessed with our weight, yet finding it harder than ever to achieve and maintain a healthy weight. Much of this is down to poor dietary advice, focusing purely on calories and exercise, with little emphasis given to the effects of when, what, and how we eat on our underlying biochemical drivers.

The idea of willpower is entrenched in dieting culture, thus locking us into battle with our body rather than working with it to give it what it needs when it needs it. Modern Western diets are littered with foods that stimulate our hunger mechanism and drive us to consume more than we need, and our inherent stops and controls have become confused. However, there is light at the end of the tunnel. Our understanding of nutrition is advancing, and we're able to implement changes to people's diets that are sustainable, relatively easy to understand and undertake, and that leave people feeling energized.

IF is a shortcut to reprogramming the body for a healthy composition. The first, very basic mechanism is that if you have fewer hours in which to eat, the likelihood is that you will eat less and hence lose weight. IF does so much more than this, however, allowing you to reset systems that could be driving weight gain without your even knowing.

### The blood sugar "roller coaster"

Our body breaks down carbohydrates into glucose to be absorbed into the bloodstream. It is then transported to cells in which the mitochondria (page 12) convert it to energy. However, we cannot store high levels of glucose in the blood, so if there's too much, the pancreas produces a hormone called insulin that signals the body to store glucose in the liver. If the liver already has a full store, the insulin converts the glucose into fatty acids that lay down deposits as adipose (fat) tissue.

Your ability to burn the fat that has been sent into storage is affected by your genetics, diet, and lifestyle choices. If this system is efficient, your body will recognize excess energy, store it as fat, and release it when needed. If it is inefficient, the body will find it harder to stimulate the release of stored fats and instead trigger the stimulus to eat more, especially driving cravings for more sugar and carbohydrates.

Carbohydrates in themselves don't make you gain weight, but too many and in the wrong forms, such as refined or white sugar, have the potential to create a vicious cycle, stimulating consumption of foods that cannot be used in real time. This is the "blood sugar roller coaster," in which too much insulin is produced to try to balance the blood sugar. IF is an effective method of retraining your insulin sensitivity and ability to burn stored fat. However, it's important to continue this work when you're in your eating window—otherwise it will be difficult for the body first to fast at all, and second to not overeat in that period. There are three simple steps to help with this:

- Reduce or avoid refined carbs (white grains, rice, bread, pasta) and switch to whole grains or brown varieties.
- Reduce or avoid sugars and sweeteners, all of which stimulate the insulin response.
- Combine carbohydrates with other food groups (protein, fat, fiber). These all reduce the time it takes for the body to break down and absorb glucose. Eating a complete meal, incorporating all the food groups, is the easiest way to balance blood sugar.

### ENCOURAGING FAT BURNING

Any weight-loss plan has to have a mechanism that drives the body to burn its fat stores. The traditional method is calorie restriction; however, this goes against biological drivers, which are telling you that you haven't eaten enough to meet your energy needs. This is where that willpower battle comes in.

Ultimately, if you want to lose weight, you have to have a calorie deficit. For losing weight and keeping it off, a daily reduction of about 500 calories is advised; any more than this can push your body toward "starvation" adaptation, in which it burns not just fat but also muscle mass. When it comes to weight loss, slow and steady wins the race.

IF makes weight loss much easier and more sustainable, working with your metabolism to slow it in order to adapt to fewer calories. Rather than constantly being in calorie deficit to induce fat-burn, the IMS and fat-burn happen in the one to four hours before you "break-fast." Then, in your eating window, you eat normally and gain energy from food. This has also been shown to have a positive effect on hormone balance, with satiation and hunger hormones better regulated in those who fast, as they naturally consume fewer calories and find it easier to lose weight and maintain a healthy body composition.

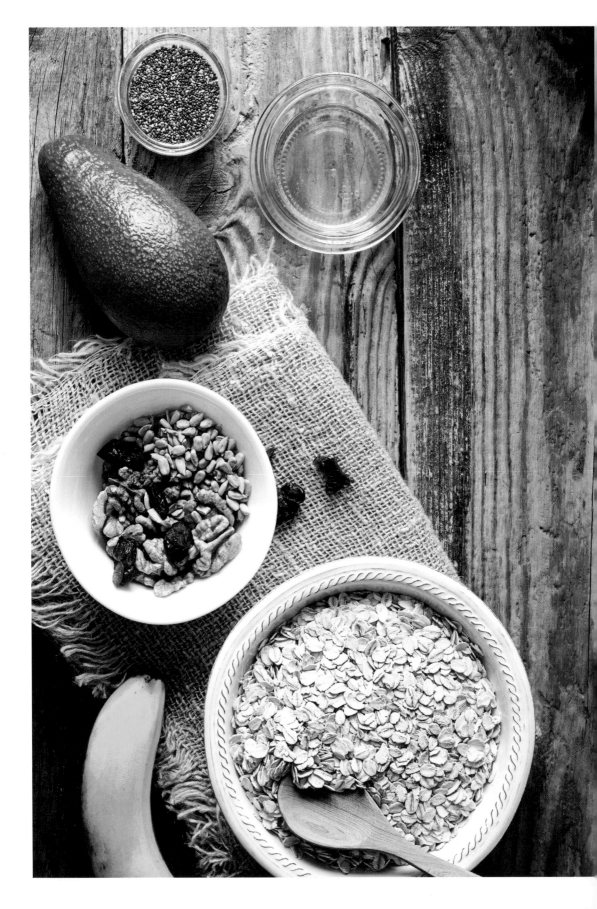

# PLANT-BASED DIET
## —The Why and the How

Whether you're looking to become fully vegan or simply leaning toward eating less meat, increasing your intake of plant-based foods is integral to both your own and the planet's health. If we all moved to at least a flexitarian-style diet, greenhouse emissions could be significantly reduced—some predict by up to half. And in terms of personal health, you have the potential to increase your daily vitality and long-term well-being simply by making a few small changes to your diet.

The principle of intermittent fasting will work with any dietary style—vegan, vegetarian, or flexitarian—but the optimal benefits can be found in combining it with a plant-based approach. As with all foods, the quality and balance of the intake is just as important as the overall principle. If you opt for plant-based but eat only processed foods, it's unlikely that you'll achieve your desired health outcome. But assuming your diet includes a high proportion of good-quality plant-based foods—including nuts, seeds, whole grains, legumes, herbs, and spices, as well as fruits and vegetables—there are a number of positive changes that you're likely to experience.

### Fiber is your friend
Fiber has been the poor relation when it comes to nutritional advice; we all know we need it, but it hasn't gotten the same focus as fats and sugars—perhaps because until recently it was seen as a nondigestible part of the diet that influenced only bowel motility. We now understand that the low levels of fiber in the standard Western diet may be a major driver of obesity, gut problems, and metabolic issues.

In the West, the average person would ideally need to raise their fiber intake by 30 percent to meet current health guidelines. In fact, to meet ancestral and non-Western diets, we should double our current intake. Increasing the plant-based element of your diet is an opportunity to easily find the extra fiber that your body needs.

### Digestion

Fiber plays a major role in gut motility and stool quality. There are two main types of fiber: soluble and nonsoluble. Nonsoluble fiber is the indigestible roughage found in abundance in plant foods. Soluble fiber is a little more elusive, although still to be found in a quality plant-based diet. The best example is the gel-like substance created by mixing chia seeds with fluids (page 114). This is soluble fiber, which works wonders inside us, enabling healthy stools to be created alongside nonsoluble fiber, thus facilitating a healthy transit that is protective of the bowel and generally makes you feel good. The digestive tract also needs fiber—particularly soluble fiber—as a source of prebiotics, to keep our healthy gut flora thriving and in balance.

Fiber exists in many different forms, depending on the plant source. The variety of these fibers is a major factor in maintaining a healthy microbiome. Therefore, the variety of plant-based foods in the diet is also important. Studies show that approximately thirty different types of plant food a week is the magic number to aim for. Remember: plant-based foods include more than simply fruits and vegetables, so thirty is actually very achievable.

## WHAT TO DO IF A HIGH-FIBER OR PLANT-BASED DIET CAUSES YOU DIGESTIVE DISCOMFORT

When increasing the plant foods in your diet, you may experience some bloating or flatulence; for most people this will settle in a few weeks as the healthy gut flora start to thrive. As both beneficial and commensal gut flora feed on prebiotics, those that cause gas as a byproduct can also benefit from increased fiber. Generally, an increase in fiber and prebiotics will help the gut flora toward a healthy balance that supports function rather than causing discomfort. If, however, your symptoms are persistent or severe, your gut flora imbalance may need some help to become optimal again, and you should consult a functional gut specialist.

A high-fiber diet can also promote weight loss. As fiber is nondigestible to humans, it takes up a lot of digestive tract space with zero calories. Yet unlike a sweetener, which also has zero calories, it stimulates our stretch receptors to feed back to our body that we're full and have eaten enough food.

### Plant-based nutrients

Plant-based foods contain a huge range of micronutrients in the form of vitamins and minerals, which are vital to maintain the thousands of biological pathways in our bodies.

Many micronutrients also double as antioxidants. Oxidative stress is the process in which cells are damaged by free radicals, as a byproduct of energy production or through environmental or dietary toxins. Free radicals are like the balls in a pinball machine, full of uncontrolled energy, smashing into anything close to them. This can cause damage to the cells or their DNA, and if left unchecked can lead to injury or illness. Antioxidants bind to free radicals, gradually neutralizing them so they're no longer problematic. Many different types of antioxidants are needed to prevent oxidative stress and cell damage—the process by which we age—and plants are a wonderful source of these.

Until recently, phytonutrients were also classed as antioxidants, working in the same way to neutralize free radicals. And for some phytonutrients, this is true: they do scavenge free radicals directly. There are others, though, such as ECGC (from green tea) and curcumin (from turmeric) that promote the antioxidative process but in a different way. Like IF, they create a hormetic effect (page 12) in the body, acting as very low-dose toxins, which create a stress response and stimulate the body's production of its own antioxidant, called glutathione. The better you are at producing glutathione, the better your liver can function and the better protected your cells are.

So, including plenty of plants in your diet is going to keep your gut healthy and reduce aging in your cells, which translates to glowing skin, an energy boost, and a reduced risk of developing disease.

## PLANT-BASED IN PRACTICE

While shifting to a plant-based diet, or simply increasing the plant foods in your regular diet, is undoubtedly a positive step for health and well-being, as the movement has grown, so has the food industry around it. As with animal food products, processed foods with lots of additives and preservatives will lack the same nutrition as foods that are prepared sensitively with quality ingredients. So the quality of your diet, in terms of raw ingredients and how food is cooked and stored, is just as important as deciding to add more plants to your diet.

In addition, if you do plan to be fully plant-based, there are a number of nutritional considerations that you need to be aware of, which are harder to achieve without animal foods. Having an understanding of how to construct a plant-based diet that gives you 100 percent of what you need and makes the most of this dietary choice is important.

Your macronutrients are the main food groups: protein, carbs, fats, and fiber. We need a balanced amount of these to create a healthy diet that fulfills both our energy and functional biological needs.

### Protein

One of the most frequently asked questions by people considering shifting to a plant-based diet or increasing the plant foods in their diet is "Where will I get my protein, and will there be enough?" Over time, the concept of the amount of protein we need has become distorted by the idea that "carbs are bad" and high-protein diets are the best way to control weight. The evidence doesn't support this: energy is provided to us from carbs and fats; protein is used for growth, repair, enzymes, and cell messaging. Plenty of plant-based foods include good levels of protein—particularly legumes, nuts and seeds, tofu and tempeh, and whole grains. Being mindful to always include at least one, or ideally two, of these food groups in a dish will enable you to have enough protein in your diet. Remember, you will also get some protein from the vegetables in your dishes, too.

### Amino acids

Proteins are made up of amino acids, and there are certain essential amino acids that we have to consume through our diet. Animal foods naturally contain all these essential amino acids in adequate amounts (they're known as complete proteins), whereas plant foods tend to contain only some of each of them (they're incomplete proteins). Food pairing is a system by which you can mix and match plant foods to expand the range of essential amino acids in a meal so as to gain all that you need. For example, pair whole grains with beans, or tofu with vegetables, or lentils with nuts (as well as many other combinations) to create enough variety to include all the essential amino acids in your plant-based diet.

## Carbohydrates

A high plant content in the diet is likely to lead to a reasonably high carb intake, but this isn't a bad thing, especially when it's combined with IF. As we've already discovered, the rate at which carbohydrates are released into the bloodstream and the efficiency of the cells in switching energy production from food-derived blood glucose to fat stores are the important factors (page 14). The recipes included in the plans are full of "good," slow-releasing complex carbs, which help with energy management and body composition.

## Fats

Over the years, fats have been tarred with the same negative nutritional connotations as carbs. In reality, we need fats to produce some hormones, to make up our cell membranes, and as an energy source. Plant-sourced fats, especially from nuts and seeds, are known as "good fats," because they're generally unsaturated. When cooking, go for fats that are already saturated or mono-unsaturated, including coconut oil, avocado oil, or olive oil. The traditional Mediterranean diet, still followed today, has always stood up to scientific investigation. The prevalence of good-quality extra virgin olive oil alongside high levels of plant-based foods is one of the main reasons it's believed to be so good for us.

## Supplements

When cutting out meat, fish, and dairy, even for a short time, you should consider supplementing some nutrients, as they will be reduced or missing completely.

Iron is found predominantly in red meat, although it does occur in plant foods, too, and this may be a nutrient that you need to supplement. Some people have a tendency toward iron anemia, which for women can be exacerbated by menstruation and pregnancy. There are also those whose bodies find it difficult to get rid of excess iron, and it is therefore important to supplement only if your iron levels are low.

Vitamin $B_{12}$ is available in the diet only via animal-based foods, including dairy. Low $B_{12}$ is also a form of anemia; signs to watch out for are low energy levels, poor concentration, and pins and needles in your feet and hands. If you're switching to a plant-based diet, it's recommended that you supplement with $B_{12}$. Unlike iron, it's a water-soluble vitamin, so you can't really overconsume it, as any excess will be excreted via the kidneys.

Fish is a rich source of essential fatty acids called omega 3s—in particular DHA and EPA— which have an extremely beneficial effect on our health. Omega 3s are also found in plant foods such as walnuts and flax, but they have to be converted to DHA and EPA, and this process isn't very efficient. Instead, it's possible to take plant-based DHA and EPA supplements that have been produced using algae rather than fish sources.

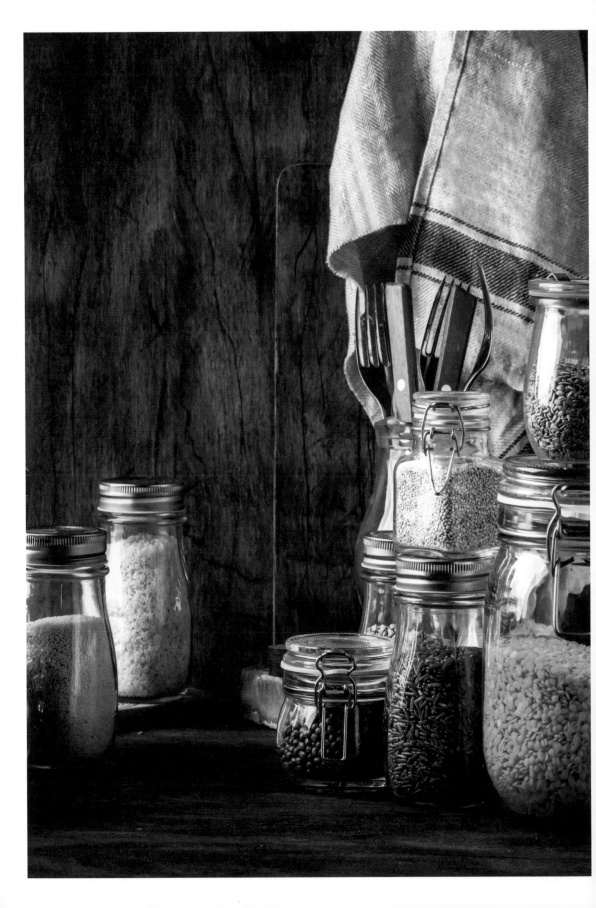

# YOUR PLANT-BASED PANTRY

In plant-based cooking, it's just as important to satisfy our taste buds as it is to support our biochemistry. Plant-based recipes create rich, deep flavor layers by using a different selection of ingredients from the ones we may be used to. To avoid amassing countless products that you'll rarely use, follow this plan for a capsule pantry of ingredients.

The two main factors to focus on when shopping are "good-quality," "plant-based" foods. With fresh foods, as much as you can, go for organic, locally sourced, seasonal products.

## SPICES

Spices are plant-based in themselves, so have their own benefits, being particularly high in phytochemicals and antioxidants.

| | |
|---|---|
| Garam masala | A spice mix originally from the Indian subcontinent, garam masala is predominantly made up of cumin and coriander seeds, along with other warming spices. |
| Ras el hanout | A great spice blend used in North African– and Middle Eastern–inspired dishes. Its name in Arabic means "head of the shop" and implies a mix of the best spices the seller has to offer. |
| Cinnamon | A warming spice, cinnamon is a great way to bring sweetness to a dish, and can be helpful in balancing blood sugar, too. |
| Smoked paprika | Its rich, smoky flavor will bring depth to a dish, with the added bonus of lots of antioxidants. |
| Turmeric | Bringing a wonderful flavor and color to a dish, turmeric is anti-inflammatory and has been shown to boost detoxification, mood, and cardiovascular health. |

## SEASONINGS

Seasonings are one of the best ways to bring deep savory or umami flavors to plant-based dishes.

| | |
|---|---|
| **Tamari** | Made from fermented soybeans, this sauce is gluten-free. If you have no issue with gluten, you can use a good-quality soy sauce. |
| **Miso paste** | A fermented soybean product with a rich umami flavor, miso paste is high in protein and nutrients. It comes in many different formulations and colors, all with slightly different flavors. White miso is the mildest. |
| **Kala namak** | Probably the most obscure seasoning used in this book. It's a salt with a high sulfur content, so it has a slightly "eggy" flavor. |
| **Nutritional yeast** | This gives a slightly cheesy flavor to plant-based dishes. It's very high in protein, so can boost the protein content of a recipe. |
| **Garlic and onion powder** | Garlic and onion powders are useful for adding flavor quickly, without the fiber and moisture of fresh onion and garlic, which can change the overall outcome of a dish. |
| **Bouillon and stocks** | Good-quality store-bought stocks are ideal and easy. Make sure you choose ones that are made from quality natural ingredients. |

## HERBS

Herbs bring another dimension to dishes. Soft, leafy herbs such as parsley, basil, cilantro, and chives are added at the end of the cooking process to give a fresh lift. Dried or woody herbs, such as thyme, oregano, and rosemary, are added at the beginning of the cooking process to infuse throughout. You can then discard the woody stems. Do your part for the planet and try growing your own to bring a touch of green to your living space and reduce carbon dioxide levels.

## DRY INGREDIENTS

Plant-based cooking requires lots of fresh fruit and vegetables, but it can also be frugal and user-friendly, as it uses lots of flours and dried and canned goods.

| | |
|---|---|
| **Legumes** | Dried pulses, peas, and lentils usually need to be soaked and cooked before using, while quality precooked versions in cans, pouches, or cartons are best for speed and convenience. From a nutritional point of view, there is little or no difference. |
| **Protein powders** | These are useful pantry ingredients, ideal for adding a protein element to smoothies, baked goods, and even soups. |
| **Gram flour** | This flour is made from garbanzo beans, so has the double benefit of being gluten-free and high in protein. |

## FRIDGE AND FREEZER

There's a myth that frozen food is of inferior quality. On the contrary: the freezing process locks in and retains nutrients.

| | |
|---|---|
| **Tofu and tempeh** | Made from fermented soybeans, these are the protein cornerstones of the plant-based diet. You can use them plain with your own marinades, or there are now many pre-marinated types available. Ideally, choose those from a non-GMO, organic source. |
| **Freezer goods** | If frozen at the source, frozen fruit and vegetables can have an advantage over their fresh counterparts, as they haven't had the chance to degrade in transit and storage. Freezer staples should include peas, corn, artichokes, berries, tropical fruits, and soybeans. |
| **Milks** | There are many milk substitutes made from nuts, grains, coconuts, and seeds. While soy milk is widely available, it's not the best form in which to consume soy, as it's not fresh or naturally fermented. Grain milks are good, as they're the most planet-friendly options. |

# DRINKS

Drinks have as many nutritional benefits as pitfalls. Our bodies don't recognize the calories in beverages: they don't make us feel full, and we don't see them as food. Yet a milky coffee, fruit juice, or soda can trigger an insulin response and easily add 100–250 calories to our daily intake. So what we drink, and when, really does matter. We should be drinking 1.5–2 liters of fluids per day, and a good proportion of that should be water.

### Caffeinated beverages

Tea and coffee contain caffeine, as well as lots of antioxidants that are good for the body. How much is advisable to drink will depend on your genetic ability to detoxify it, but whether you're a fast or slow detoxifier, tea and coffee should be taken black during the fast, with no sugar or sweeteners. Alternatives include green tea and matcha green tea. They contain caffeine and antioxidants that are good for your liver and that promote fat-burning, but also a calming component called L-theanine.

### Alcohol, sodas, and fruit juice

Sodas and alcohol contain completely hollow calories with known health drawbacks, so should be avoided completely while on the plan. Fruit juices are often marketed as healthy alternatives, but even from "natural sources" the sugar will still cause an insulin spike, so it's advised to keep these drinks to a minimum.

## HERBAL TEAS

Herbal teas generally don't contain any caffeine but do contain healing herbs and spices. Here are a few to look out for:

*Ginger* soothes the digestive tract and helps gastric motility
*Dandelion* stimulates digestion, especially of fats
*Fennel* aids digestion, relieving bloating and stomach cramps
*Camomile* helps relaxation
*Peppermint* relaxes muscles (avoid if you suffer from indigestion or reflux)
*Lemon Balm* reduces anxiety and boosts cognitive function

A plant-based drink with good quality matcha or beneficial spices such as turmeric and ginger can be a healthy and comforting addition to your daily plan.

## Matcha Latte

SERVES 1 | 120 cal

¾ cup oat milk

½ teaspoon premium-grade matcha powder

**1.** Pour a splash of the milk into a cup and add the matcha. Stir to dissolve the powder into a paste.

**2.** Heat the rest of the milk to your desired latte temperature, making sure it doesn't boil. Pour the warmed milk into the cup with the matcha paste, stir well, and serve.

## Golden Latte

SERVES 1 | 160 cal

1 cup coconut milk, in a carton (or any plant-based milk)

⅛ teaspoon ground turmeric

¼ teaspoon ground cinnamon

⅛ teaspoon ground ginger

pinch of black pepper

**1.** Place the coconut milk and spices in a saucepan over low heat and allow the spices to infuse for 10 minutes. Pour into a mug to serve.

## DESIGNING YOUR FASTING AND EATING WINDOWS

IF can make changes to our underlying biochemistry that help us manage our daily and long-term health, focus, and energy levels, and create a healthy body composition. There are, however, potential slipups along the way that can easily undo our best intentions. Use the following steps to get the most out of your IF plan.

Everyone is going to need different fast and eat windows. Our livers have differing abilities to store glycogen, and therefore the point at which we make our glucose-to-ketone switch will be different for everyone. Equally, the current number and health of our mitochondria, as well as our insulin sensitivity, will have an impact. Fasting for too long too soon could have a counterproductive effect.

The sixteen-hour fast with an eight-hour eating window is often seen as an achievable daily routine that fits in with the average person's commitments. A fast of twenty hours with a four-hour eating window is generally seen as the maximum for daily fasting.

If you're new to IF, it might be best to start with a twelve- to thirteen-hour fast and gradually build your fasting period toward sixteen hours. If the short fast feels easy, then build up over a few days. If you feel any of the following symptoms—headache, dizziness, faintness, brain fog, sweating, tingling lips, shakiness or trembling, racing heart or palpitations—you are not effectively switching to ketones and should shorten the fast period. Otherwise you will be pushing your body into a stressed low blood sugar state, which will have a negative effect. After a few weeks, once IF has started to work on your underlying metabolism, you can build up your fast time in half-hour increments.

It's also important to align your fast with your circadian rhythm. This means that you should fast overnight while you sleep, breaking your fast at lunchtime and allowing for the traditional social interaction of the evening meal. On the other hand, if you wanted your eating window to be earlier in the day—for example, 8:00 a.m. to 4:00 p.m.—you would reap the same benefits. It's really up to you; whatever works for your body and your life.

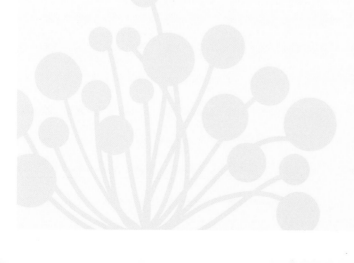

## MEAL STRUCTURING AND DIETARY CHOICES

You are going to be hungriest at your "break-fast" meal, so it's important to eat something that will satiate you. The calorie-cutting culture has, over the years, continued to diminish both the quantity and quality of our breakfasts. Whether you're following an IF plan or not, what you choose at that first meal of the day has a huge influence on your remaining dietary choices for the rest of the day. It's at this meal more than all the others that you should find balance and abundance on your plate by combining complex carbohydrates, fiber, protein, and fats. For effective blood sugar balance, while you're in your eating window, this same full spectrum of macronutrients at every meal is ideal.

If you're aiming for optimal health without any particular weight loss goal (page 35), you can simply compress your regular three-meal structure into your eight-hour eating window. If you're aiming for weight loss (page 53), integrating the 500-calorie deficit can be done by replacing your late lunch with a mini meal. And banish the idea of snacks—every meal is a meal that should count.

Fasting is not only important to reset our metabolic health, it also plays a vital role in our gut health. Ideally, you should have a twelve-hour gap between your meals overnight, and roughly four hours between your daytime meals. In turn, poor digestive function plays a role in fatigue, immune issues, mood, and brain health.

### IS IF FOR EVERYONE?

Every healthy person should aim to have a twelve-hour overnight fast. However, there are those for whom fasting is not advised as a dietary intervention. For anyone in the following groups, please seek medical advice and monitoring for any diet and lifestyle change.

- Those with a diagnosis of diabetes.
- Those on medication that may be affected by changes to the frequency of eating.
- Pregnant women.
- Those with a history of eating disorders.

# EXERCISE

By using exercise in combination with IF, it's possible to enhance your results further. Exercise is another method of making your body switch from glucose to ketone burning. Ideally, you want to schedule exercise after your body has switched to ketone fat burning, toward the end of your fast and before you have your "break-fast" meal. If you have an efficient switch and healthy mitochondria, you shouldn't have any difficulty completing your normal exercise regimen. If you feel that you're struggling, this would indicate that you're pushing a positive hormetic effect into a counterproductive state. If this is the case, try moving your exercise and breakfast a little earlier.

**What exercise should I do?**

If you already have an exercise routine, you can easily integrate it into your day while on the plan. If you don't exercise at all, then it's important to think about getting moving. Like our dietary needs, preferences, and goals, we're all individuals, so there's no one-size-fits-all in terms of the exercise you should do. The most important thing is to move, and move regularly; evidence shows that a sedentary lifestyle is just not good for us. It doesn't have to be organized exercise, however: walking, gardening, and cleaning all count.

If you have a specific goal in terms of body composition, there are different exercises that can help you achieve that. High intensity interval training (HIIT) is great for weight loss; resistance exercise uses weights for building muscle; and Pilates and yoga build flexibility and core strength. Team sports are a great way to socialize while getting fit, and signing up for a challenge, such as a 10k run, is a good way to stay motivated.

Spend some time thinking about what you want to get out of your exercise, aside from the fitness; try a few new things and see what works for you. You will have weeks when it feels good and you enjoy it and other weeks when it feels like a chore, but making exercise a habit, just like changing your eating habits, is the best way for it to become integrated into your everyday life over time.

*When it comes to IF and nutrition in general, more is not necessarily better. Finding the "sweet spot" that works for you should be your aim. Always listen to your body; it will guide you toward the best strategy and balance.*

# CONSCIOUS EATING

Our busy modern lives mean that we often don't make time to sit down and enjoy a meal; we eat on the run or at our desks, distracted by our phones or TV. This has a negative effect on our mood and digestive health, and therefore our overall well-being.

Wolfing down food without thought often leads to less chewing. Chewing stimulates digestive enzyme production and breaks down the food so it can be absorbed optimally. Without it, the likelihood of digestive problems increases, and the nutrients you get from your food may be reduced. Stress is also counterproductive to a healthy digestive system.

## FIVE EASY STEPS TO HEALTHIER MEALTIMES

Reclaiming your mealtimes is such a small step, but will have a significant impact on your well-being, as well as your productivity, focus, and efficiency.

1. **Be mindful of your hunger mechanism.** Prepare and eat food when your body needs it. Take time to plan and make meals. This will connect you to your food, helping you appreciate it as both fuel and pleasure.

2. **Make time to eat.** Set aside thirty minutes for every meal, even if it doesn't take that long. Give your body time to savor your food and time to let it all go down.

3. **Choose a pleasant and relaxing environment in which to eat.** That may be a dinner table, but could also be out in nature—on a park bench, for example.

4. **Eat with no distractions apart from friends, family, and colleagues.** Eat some meals alone and some with other people. Enjoy the social aspect, but sometimes just focus on the taste and texture of the food.

5. **For every mouthful you take, chew forty times;** it takes only a few seconds.

# ALL YOU NEED TO KNOW

*Will I be hungry?*
If you're new to fasting, you're likely to be hungry during the fasting period. Building up your fasting window over time can help your body transition without hunger becoming overwhelming. It's important to recognize the difference between feeling hungry (thinking about food, rumbly stomach, etc.) and low blood sugar (poor focus, shaky, nausea, faint). If you're experiencing the latter, you're fasting for too long and need to adjust your timing. During your eating window you should be eating enough to feel satiated.

*Is there anything I shouldn't eat?*
Avoid processed foods full of additives, unhealthy fats, and foods that lack nutrients.

*How long can I fast for?*
You can fast for as long as it's healthy for your body to do so. The plans provided are designed for the most common timing of sixteen hours of fasting. Listen to your body and adjust the plan to suit you.

*Do the plans fit with full-time work?*
Yes. If working properly, the fasting period should provide increased focus and energy. A batch-and-freeze strategy is important for maintaining a healthy diet when you have a busy life.

*What happens if I miss a day?*
It doesn't matter if you miss a day. The benefits of intermittent fasting aren't wiped out by a "day off." For the long term, it's recommended that you find a level of integration that works for you and your social life. Regularity and sustainability are key to dietary strategies more so than extreme adherence.

*Can I eat out while doing the plan?*
Yes, you can eat out. If you follow the dietary advice given to inform your ordering, then great! If it's not possible, don't worry; tomorrow is another day.

*Is there an optimal time to start? Do you need to be mentally fit and healthy? Do you need to do any physical or mental preparation?*
You can increase the amount of plant-based foods in your diet anytime. As IF works on the principle of hormesis (page 11), it's best to start when you aren't feeling ill. Gradually build up your fast window, as you are less likely to overstress your body that way.

# STARTING THE PLAN

Take some time to prepare before starting the plan. Analyze the plan you've selected and make sure it will fit into your life and work schedule for the next two weeks. Consider how long it will take you to shop for and prepare food, where you will be eating, and which recipes you like and don't like. With these things in mind, make any changes to the plan that you need to, and create a shopping list of ingredients. The Plant-Based Pantry (pages 23–25) contains a list of staples that you can buy in advance and that will keep throughout the plan. For the fresh produce, it's best to shop at the start of Week 1 and Week 2; try to buy local, seasonal, and organic wherever possible.

### During the plan

Listen to your body. Don't try to push it too far, especially with regards to fasting and eating windows. While it's normal to feel hungry toward the end of the fast period, you should not feel overly tired or unfocused. You shouldn't feel hungry once your fast is broken and you're in your eating window. If you do, increase your portion size slightly at mealtimes, and try playing around with the eating times. For example, if you're breaking fast at 11:00 a.m. but getting very hungry in the early evening and a 7:00 p.m. dinnertime seems like a stretch, move your dinner to 6:00 p.m. Be sure to stay hydrated and look after yourself while following the plan, and get enough sleep and relaxation.

If you feel you're in need of something sweet while on the plan, cherries and chocolate are an instant healthy dessert that's high in antioxidants. Once or twice a week, during your eating window, you could add either two squares of dark chocolate plus $^2/_3$ cup frozen or thawed cherries *or* a portion of fruit. Choose good-quality fair-trade chocolate with at least 70 percent cocoa solids. A portion of fruit could be 1 apple, $^2/_3$ cup berries, 1 banana, or 1 kiwi fruit, for example. Always eat fruit whole and as part of a meal. You could also add an extra Matcha or Golden Latte (page 27) once or twice a week within your eating window.

### Finishing the plan

Well done! I hope by now you will have discovered your ideal eating and fasting windows, finding the "sweet spot" that triggers the shift to fat-burning without low blood sugar stress. IF is a strategy that you should always employ to some degree, establishing a minimum twelve-hour overnight fast as standard, and going forward, I hope you'll integrate some of the new recipes into your weekly meal plans. Adding more plant-based foods to your diet is a positive step toward improving your own health and that of the environment.

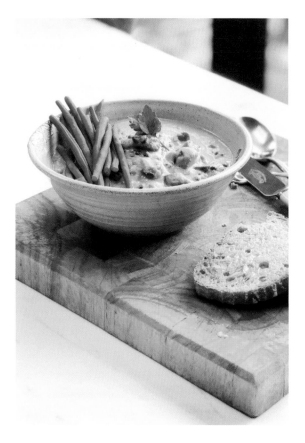

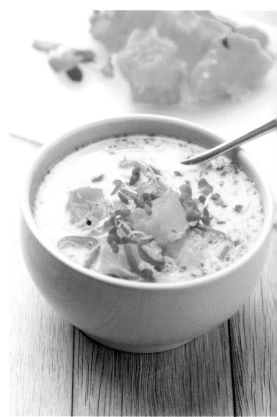

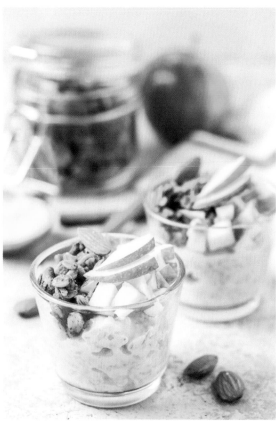

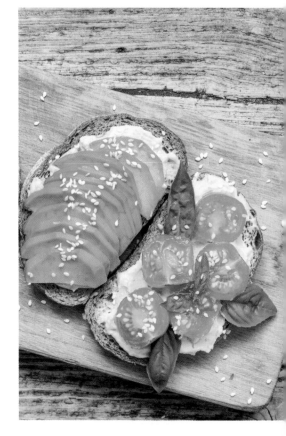

# 14-Day Meal Plan
## Optimal Health

---

This plan is designed to boost health and maintain weight, with an average of 2000 calories per day, while reaping the benefits of a plant-based diet and time-restricted eating.

Most of the dishes are interchangeable, meaning that if you're strapped for time, you can batch cook and either refrigerate or freeze for use on another day. And if you need to take a packed lunch to work, you can choose the dishes that are most practical for this. Lastly, choose the dishes that you like the sound of, that excite your taste buds; food should be as much about enjoyment as health.

# WEEK 1

# DAY 1

First day of the plan; hopefully you're prepared both practically and mentally. It's easier than you think. Ease yourself in by starting with a fast of thirteen or fourteen hours.

## 7–8 a.m.
Black coffee or green tea

## 9–10 a.m.
Scrambled tofu *(page 88)*
Matcha Latte *(page 27)*

## 2–3 p.m.
Peaches and spiced garbanzo beans with
arugula dressing *(page 97)*

## 7 p.m.
Butternut laksa bowl *(page 120)*

# DAY 2

Today, extend your fasting window to fourteen to fifteen hours. Remember, it's normal to feel hungry, especially toward the end of the fast, but you should still feel alert and energized. You're looking for the "sweet spot" where you shift to fat-burning without causing low blood sugar symptoms.

### 7–8 a.m.
Black coffee or green tea

### 10–11 a.m.
Chickpea omelet mushrooms *(page 87)*
Green or herbal tea

### 3–4 p.m.
Vegan Caesar Salad *(page 101)*

### 7 p.m.
Beet burger *(page 126)*

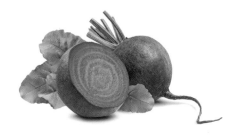

# DAY 3

If you found that yesterday's fasting window was easily doable, extend it further to fifteen to sixteen hours. If you have time today, look ahead and see if there are some dishes you can prepare in advance. Make a soup or batch cook for another day, for example.

### 7–8 a.m.
Black coffee or green tea

### 10–11 a.m.
Green or herbal tea

### 12 p.m.
Apple, almond, and cinnamon overnight oats *(page 74)*

### 3–4 p.m.
Butternut, macadamia, and sage soup *(page 104)*

### 7 p.m.
Olive, herb, and lemon vegetable casserole *(page 124)*

# DAY 4

I hope you've found your ideal eating and fasting window by now. The plan is based on the classic 16:8 format, but you can continue to adjust the timing to work for you.

### 7–8 a.m.
Black coffee or green tea

### 10–11 a.m.
Green or herbal tea

### 12 p.m.
Mushrooms, pine nuts, and arugula on rye bread *(page 83)*

### 3–4 p.m.
Buckwheat noodle, seaweed, asparagus, and edamame salad *(page 98)*

### 7 p.m.
Quick pita "pizza" with homemade pesto *(page 125)*

# DAY 5

Hump day! Your body will still be getting used to the fasting, so the feeling of hunger in the mornings may seem to last a long time. Persevere for a few more days; you'll start to adapt, and it will seem easier.

### 7–8 a.m.
Black coffee or green tea

### 10–11 a.m.
Green or herbal tea

### 12 p.m.
Very berry protein smoothie *(page 80)*

### 3–4 p.m.
Roasted carrot and lentil salad *(page 94)*

### 7 p.m.
Vegan mushroom and Puy lentil stroganoff *(page 134)*

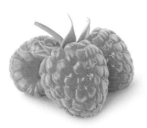

# DAY 6

If you haven't already, start to think about incorporating exercise or movement into your daily routine. Combined with the fasting, it will work to maximize your IMS (page 12).

### 7–8 a.m.
Black coffee or green tea

### 10–11 a.m.
Green or herbal tea

### 12 p.m.
Black pepper cashew "cream cheese" and fruit toast *(page 76)*

### 3–4 p.m.
Roasted artichoke, white bean, and tomato salad *(page 100)*

### 7 p.m.
Pineapple, peanut, and vegetable curry *(page 138)*

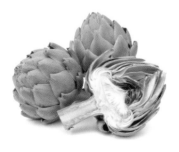

# DAY 7

Well done! Week one is complete, and you should be settling into your new routine. Reward yourself tonight with some self-care relaxation: maybe watch an uplifting movie or run yourself a candlelit bath and relax with an extra Golden Latte (page 27).

## 7–8 a.m.
Black coffee or green tea

## 10–11 a.m.
Green or herbal tea

## 12 p.m.
Tempeh "bacon" BLT *(page 78)*

## 3–4 p.m.
Watercress, basil, and almond soup *(page 96)*

## 7 p.m.
Mexican black beans with guacamole *(page 130)*

# WEEK 2

# DAY 8

Think about using the morning to do something positive to keep you busy. Maybe try a new exercise or yoga class, or tackle that cupboard that needs clearing out. Maybe invite some friends or family over to enjoy your "break-fast" as a social brunch.

### 7–8 a.m.
Black coffee or green tea

### 10–11 a.m.
Green or herbal tea

### 12 p.m.
Corn and zucchini fritters with salsa *(page 86)*
Golden Latte *(page 27)*

### 3–4 p.m.
Peaches and spiced garbanzo beans with
arugula dressing *(page 97)*

### 7 p.m.
Sweet potato and spinach dal *(page 122)*

# DAY 9

Use today as a prep day for the week ahead. Revisit the plan to make any tweaks you think necessary: think about any lessons you learned in the previous week, your eating and fasting windows, how much time you have to cook and prepare meals, and your upcoming commitments.

## 7–8 a.m.
Black coffee or green tea

## 10–11 a.m.
Green or herbal tea

## 12 p.m.
Coconut French toast with cherry compote *(page 82)*

Matcha Latte *(page 27)*

## 3–4 p.m.
Vegan Caesar Salad *(page 101)*

## 7 p.m.
Vegan cauliflower "cheese" with smoky

mushrooms *(page 136)*

# DAY 10

Hopefully your body and mind are getting used to your new IF routine. You should be feeling less hungry and finding it easier to sustain without thinking too much about it. Everything on today's menu can be batch-cooked, frozen, and stored for another day or another week.

### 7–8 a.m.
Black coffee or green tea

### 10–11 a.m.
Green or herbal tea

### 12 p.m.
Walnut and banana bread *(page 90)*

### 3–4 p.m.
Butternut, macadamia, and sage soup *(page 104)*

### 7 p.m.
Porcini mushroom and thyme speltotto *(page 140)*

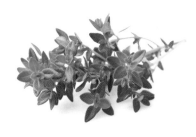

# DAY 11

This plant-based diet has most likely increased your intake of fiber. While this should be good for your system, if your gut flora is out of balance, it may cause symptoms such as gas and bloating. Try some probiotic supplements or seek advice from a professional to help rebalance it.

## 7–8 a.m.
Black coffee or green tea

## 10–11 a.m.
Green or herbal tea

## 12 p.m.
Crushed creamy basil chili peas on toast *(page 91)*

## 3–4 p.m.
Buckwheat noodle, seaweed, asparagus, and edamame salad *(page 98)*

## 7 p.m.
Fennel, leek, and pea baked barley *(page 133)*

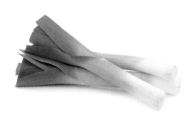

# DAY 12

What movement have you done this week? Do you have space today to incorporate some more? Perhaps you could walk part of the way to work, or take a walking meeting rather than sitting down indoors.

## 7–8 a.m.

Black coffee or green tea

## 10–11 a.m.

Green or herbal tea

## 12 p.m.

Pina-kale-ada protein smoothie *(page 80)*

## 3–4 p.m.

Roasted carrot and lentil salad *(page 94)*

## 7 p.m.

Special fried cauliflower and quinoa "rice" *(page 129)*

# DAY 13

Are you missing animal products in your diet? It's good to think about what you feel you need both physically and psychologically. Completely eliminating something can often make you crave what you can't have, so it's good to think about how you can make sustainable changes.

### 7–8 a.m.
Black coffee or green tea

### 10–11 a.m.
Green or herbal tea

### 12 p.m.
Banana and peanut butter oatmeal *(page 77)*

### 3–4 p.m.
Italian white bean and cavolo nero soup *(page 102)*

### 7 p.m.
Eggplant with miso tahini glaze and
sesame cucumber *(page 128)*

# DAY 14

Well done on completing the fourteen-day plan! I hope it's been an enjoyable learning curve, both in the kitchen and connecting with your body. Don't worry if you didn't manage to do every day or every recipe; these strategies don't need to be applied 100 percent of the time to be beneficial.

### 7–8 a.m.
Black coffee or green tea

### 10–11 a.m.
Green or herbal tea

### 12 p.m.
Hummus, avocado, and tomato toast *(page 84)*

### 3–4 p.m.
Watercress, basil, and almond soup *(page 96)*

### 7 p.m.
Vegan ragu *(page 132)*

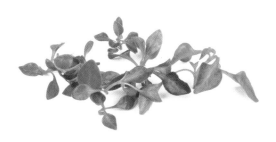

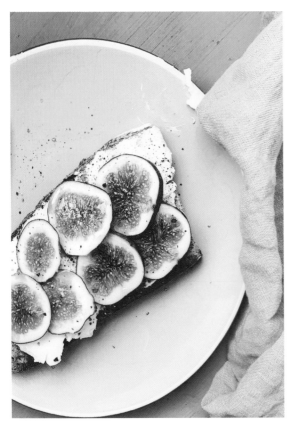

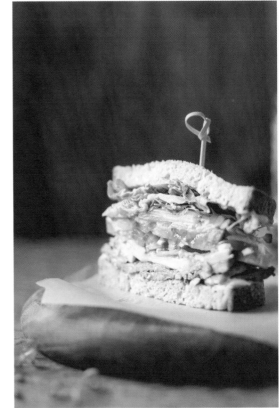

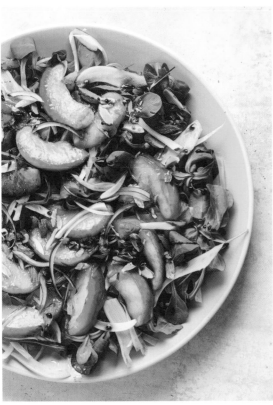

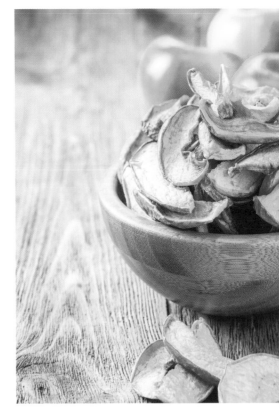

## *14-Day Meal Plan*
# Optimal Weight Loss

---

This plan is designed to start a sustainable weight-loss journey, with an average of 1200–1500 calories per day, while still reaping the health benefits of a plant-based diet and time-restricted eating.

Most of the dishes are interchangeable, meaning that if you're strapped for time, you can batch cook and either refrigerate or freeze for use on another day. And if you need to take a packed lunch to work, you can choose the dishes that are most practical for this.

The afternoon meal (3–4 p.m.) is a mini meal. The idea of a "snack" has been linked to overeating, so renaming these dishes "mini meals" is the best way to change perspective and include them as part of the daily calorie count.

# WEEK 1

# DAY 1

First day of the plan; hopefully you're prepared both practically and mentally. It's easier than you think. Ease yourself in by starting with a fast of thirteen to fourteen hours.

### 7–8 a.m.
Black coffee or green tea

### 9–10 a.m.
Scrambled tofu *(page 88)*

Green or herbal tea

### 3–4 p.m.
Summer rolls with satay sauce *(page 110)*

### 7 p.m.
Butternut laksa bowl *(page 120)*

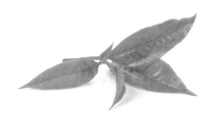

# DAY 2

Today, extend your fasting window to fourteen to fifteen hours. Remember, it's normal to feel hungry, especially toward the end of the fast, but you should still feel alert and energized. You're looking for the "sweet spot" where you shift to fat-burning without causing low blood sugar symptoms.

## 7–8 a.m.
Black coffee or green tea

## 10–11 a.m.
Chickpea omelet mushrooms *(page 87)*

Green or herbal tea

## 3–4 p.m.
Muhammara with crudités (bell pepper and walnut dip) *(page 113)*

## 7 p.m.
Beet burger *(page 126)*

# DAY 3

If you found that yesterday's fasting window was easily doable, extend it further to fifteen to sixteen hours. If you have time today, look ahead and see if there are some dishes you can prepare in advance. Make a soup or batch cook for another day, for example.

### 7–8 a.m.
Black coffee or green tea

### 10–11 a.m.
Green or herbal tea

### 12 p.m.
Apple, almond, and cinnamon overnight oats *(page 74)*

### 3–4 p.m.
Tamari cashews *(page 109)*

### 7 p.m.
Olive, herb, and lemon vegetable casserole *(page 124)*

# DAY 4

I hope you've found your ideal eating and fasting window by now. The plan is based on the classic 16:8 format, but you can continue to adjust the timing to work for you.

### 7–8 a.m.

Black coffee or green tea

### 10–11 a.m.

Green or herbal tea

### 12 p.m.

Mushrooms, pine nuts, and arugula on rye bread *(page 83)*

### 3–4 p.m.

Cherry almond chia bowl *(page 114)*

### 7 p.m.

Quick pita "pizza" with homemade pesto *(page 125)*

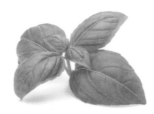

# DAY 5

Hump day! Your body will still be getting used to the fasting, so the feeling of hunger in the mornings may seem to last a long time. Persevere for a few more days; you'll start to adapt, and it will seem easier.

## 7–8 a.m.
Black coffee or green tea

## 10–11 a.m.
Green or herbal tea

## 12 p.m.
Very berry protein smoothie *(page 80)*

## 3–4 p.m.
Apple cinnamon chips with peanut butter *(page 116)*

## 7 p.m.
Vegan mushroom and Puy lentil stroganoff *(page 134)*

# DAY 6

If you haven't already, start to think about incorporating exercise or movement into your daily routine. Combined with the fasting, it will work to maximize your IMS (page 12).

### 7–8 a.m.
Black coffee or green tea

### 10–11 a.m.
Green or herbal tea

### 12 p.m.
Black pepper cashew "cream cheese"
and fruit toast *(page 76)*

### 3–4 p.m.
Walnut and mushroom pâté *(page 112)*

### 7 p.m.
Pineapple, peanut, and vegetable curry *(page 138)*

# DAY 7

Well done! Week one is complete, and you should be settling into your new routine. Reward yourself tonight with some self-care relaxation: maybe watch an uplifting movie or run yourself a candlelit bath.

### 7–8 a.m.
Black coffee or green tea

### 10–11 a.m.
Green or herbal tea

### 12 p.m.
Tempeh "bacon" BLT *(page 78)*

### 3–4 p.m.
Matcha power ball *(page 108)*

### 7 p.m.
Mexican black beans with guacamole *(page 130)*

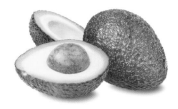

# WEEK 2

# DAY 8

Think about using the morning to do something positive to keep you busy. Maybe try a new exercise or yoga class, or tackle that cupboard that needs clearing out. Maybe invite some friends or family over to enjoy your "break-fast" as a social brunch.

### 7–8 a.m.
Black coffee or green tea

### 10–11 a.m.
Green or herbal tea

### 12 p.m.
Corn and zucchini fritters with salsa *(page 86)*

### 3–4 p.m.
Summer rolls with satay sauce *(page 110)*

### 7 p.m.
Sweet potato and spinach dal *(page 122)*

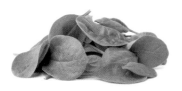

# DAY 9

Use today as a prep day for the week ahead. Revisit the plan to make any tweaks you think necessary: think about any lessons you learned in the previous week, your eating and fasting windows, how much time you have to cook and prepare meals, and your upcoming commitments.

### 7–8 a.m.

Black coffee or green tea

### 10–11 a.m.

Green or herbal tea

### 12 p.m.

Coconut French toast with cherry compote *(page 82)*

### 3–4 p.m.

Muhammara with crudités (bell pepper and walnut dip) *(page 113)*

### 7 p.m.

Vegan cauliflower "cheese" with smoky mushrooms *(page 136)*

# DAY 10

Hopefully your body and mind are getting used to your new IF routine.
You should be feeling less hungry and finding it easier to sustain without
thinking too much about it. Both the banana bread and speltotto can be
batch-cooked, frozen, and stored for another day or another week.

### 7–8 a.m.

Black coffee or green tea

### 10–11 a.m.

Green or herbal tea

### 12 p.m.

Walnut and banana bread *(page 90)*

### 3–4 p.m.

Apple cinnamon chips with peanut butter *(page 116)*

### 7 p.m.

Porcini mushroom and thyme speltotto *(page 140)*

# DAY 11

This plant-based diet has most likely increased your intake of fiber. While this should be good for your system, if your gut flora is out of balance, it may cause symptoms such as gas and bloating. Try some probiotic supplements or seek advice from a professional to help rebalance it.

### 7–8 a.m.
Black coffee or green tea

### 10–11 a.m.
Green or herbal tea

### 12 p.m.
Crushed creamy basil chili peas on toast *(page 91)*

### 3–4 p.m.
Cherry almond chia bowl *(page 114)*

### 7 p.m.
Fennel, leek, and pea baked barley *(page 133)*

# DAY 12

What movement have you done this week? Do you have space today to incorporate some more? Perhaps you could walk part of the way to work, or take a walking meeting rather than sitting down indoors.

### 7–8 a.m.
Black coffee or green tea

### 10–11 a.m.
Green or herbal tea

### 12 p.m.
Pina-kale-ada protein smoothie *(page 80)*

### 3–4 p.m.
Tamari cashews *(page 109)*

### 7 p.m.
Special fried cauliflower and quinoa "rice" *(page 129)*

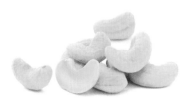

# DAY 13

Are you missing animal products in your diet? It's good to think about what you feel you need both physically and psychologically. Completely eliminating something can often make you crave what you can't have, so it's good to think about how you can make sustainable changes.

### 7–8 a.m.

Black coffee or green tea

### 10–11 a.m.

Green or herbal tea

### 12 p.m.

Banana and peanut butter oatmeal *(page 77)*

### 3–4 p.m.

Walnut and mushroom pâté *(page 112)*

### 7 p.m.

Eggplant with miso tahini glaze and

sesame cucumber *(page 128)*

# DAY 14

Well done on completing the fourteen-day plan! I hope it's been an enjoyable learning curve, both in the kitchen and connecting with your body. Don't worry if you didn't manage to do every day or every recipe; these strategies don't need to be applied 100 percent of the time to be beneficial.

## 7–8 a.m.

Black coffee or green tea

## 10–11 a.m.

Green or herbal tea

## 12 p.m.

Hummus, avocado, and tomato toast *(page 84)*

## 3–4 p.m.

Matcha power ball *(page 108)*

## 7 p.m.

Vegan ragu *(page 132)*

# RECIPES

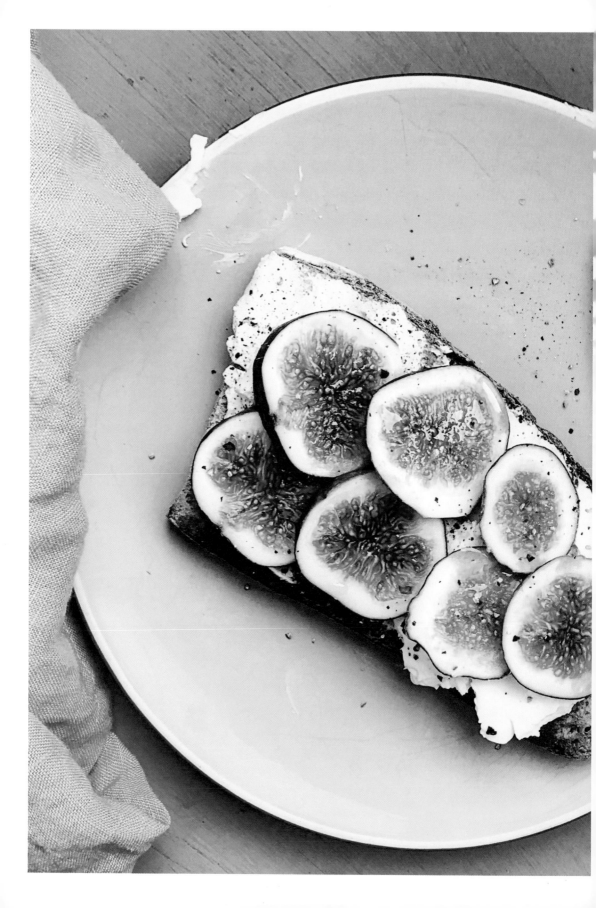

# Breakfast

---

The old nutritional adage that "breakfast is the most important meal of the day" still holds true, even when you aren't eating it at the traditional time. What's important is that it has the right nutritional makeup to give you sustained energy, keeping you feeling fuller for longer. This means a combination of proteins, fibers, complex carbohydrates, and healthy fats. The following recipes are all designed with that knowledge in mind: breaking the fast with nutritional balance so that you feel energized in the short term and so the body is nourished in the long term.

*Black pepper cashew "cream cheese" and fruit toast (page 76)*

# APPLE, ALMOND, AND CINNAMON OVERNIGHT OATS

SERVES 1 | **Prep time:** 5 minutes, plus overnight refrigeration
**Nutrition per serving:** 479 cal | 15.6g protein | 59.6g carbs | 22g fat | 10.4g fiber

*Overnight oats are a quick, simple, and portable breakfast. The only tricky thing about this recipe is remembering to prepare it the night before. It can also be made in larger batches for convenience, as it will last for two to three days in the refrigerator. Passion fruit and coconut milk also work well as a tropical alternative.*

½ apple

½ cup (1½ ounces) rolled oats

⅓ cup (1 ounce) ground
  almonds

⅓ cup oat milk

⅓ cup apple juice

½ teaspoon cinnamon

pinch of sea salt

**1.** Grate the apple into a bowl or jar, then add all the other ingredients and mix well.

**2.** Cover the bowl with plastic wrap or seal the jar and store in the refrigerator overnight, ready for an instant breakfast the following morning.

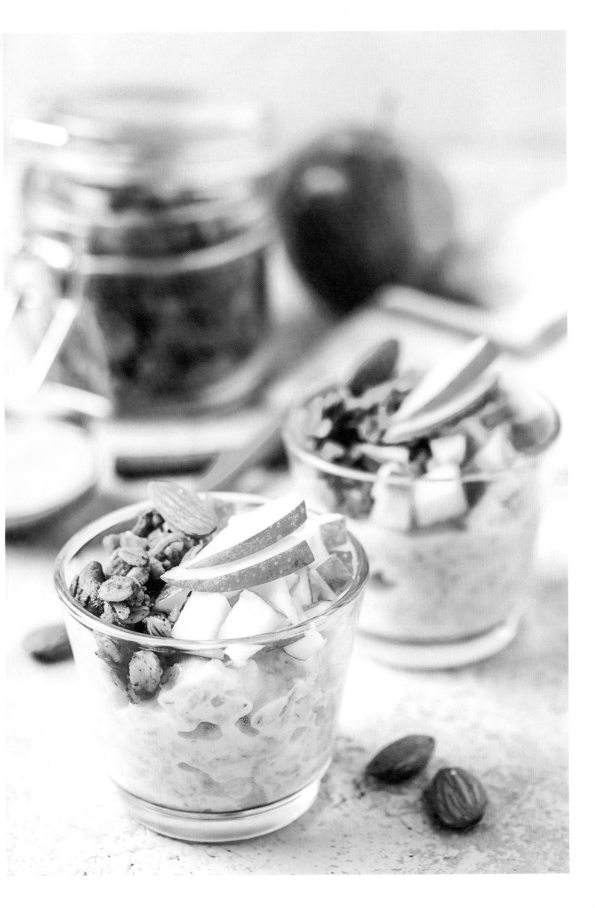

# BLACK PEPPER CASHEW "CREAM CHEESE" AND FRUIT TOAST

SERVES 1 | **Prep time:** 5 minutes, plus 2 hours' soaking (or overnight) | **Cook time:** 2 minutes
Nutrition per serving: 377 cal | 10g protein | 46g carbs | 18g fat | 9g fiber

*Nuts are so much more than a minor ingredient in baking or a healthy snack option. Cashews are creamy, so they work particularly well as a plant-based cheese alternative. The combination of black pepper and fruit may be a new flavor pairing to you, but it's one that will make your taste buds sing.*

*For the black pepper cashew "cheese":*

1⅓ cups raw cashew nuts

juice of ½ lemon

2 tablespoons nutritional yeast

1 tablespoon water

pinch of sea salt

ground black pepper

1 slice of whole grain bread (try a dark rye), toasted

1 fig or 3 strawberries or 1 peach

**1.** Place the cashew nuts in water and soak for at least 2 hours, or (ideally) overnight.

**2.** Drain and rinse the cashews, then place them in a food processor with all the other cashew "cheese" ingredients and pulse for 5–10 minutes to blend. Be patient with it, continually stopping to scrape the mixture from the sides of the bowl before pulsing again until smooth. Taste, and add more black pepper if you like.

**3.** To assemble the fruit toast, spread a little of the cashew "cheese" over the toasted bread. Add slices of your desired fruit—ideally one that's in season, or you could use a compote of frozen fruits, which can be used all year round. Crack a little more freshly ground black pepper over the top to serve.

# BANANA AND PEANUT BUTTER OATMEAL

SERVES 1 | **Prep time:** 5 minutes | **Cook time:** 15 minutes
**Nutrition per serving:** 520 cal | 16.5g protein | 62.6g carbs | 22g fat | 11.1g fiber

*Who doesn't love the classic combination of banana and peanut butter? It's ideal for those days when you need a hug in a bowl. Cooking the oats with the banana means that they're sweetened using only whole natural fruit. Also, pick your peanut butter carefully: choose one without added oils, sugars, or sweeteners.*

1 banana

½ cup (1½ ounces) rolled oats

scant ⅔ cup water

scant ⅔ cup oat milk

good pinch of sea salt

2 tablespoons crunchy peanut
  butter

**1.** Slice the banana into a saucepan, then add the oats, water, oat milk, and salt. Bring to a boil, then reduce the heat and simmer, stirring regularly, for around 15 minutes, until the oats are cooked through and the oatmeal has thickened.

**2.** Remove from the heat and stir in the peanut butter until well combined. Serve immediately.

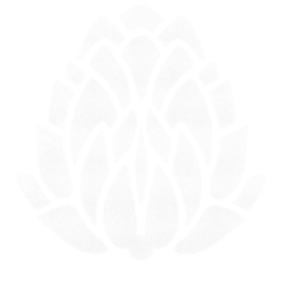

# TEMPEH "BACON" BLT

SERVES 1 | **Prep time:** 10 minutes | **Cook time:** 5 minutes
Nutrition per serving: 691 cal | 28.5g protein | 63g carbs | 34.4g fat | 10.9g fiber

*This tasty sandwich, rich in smoky and umami flavors, is a pretty epic way to break your fast. It feels incredibly indulgent but is really just full of the good stuff. Made from fermented soybeans, tempeh has a higher content of protein, dietary fiber, and vitamins and is easier to digest.*

2 slices of whole grain bread
   (try spelt or rye sourdough)
½ tablespoon vegan
   mayonnaise (optional)
¼ avocado, sliced
1 tomato, sliced
pinch of sea salt and ground
black pepper
1 baby gem lettuce leaf

*For the tempeh "bacon":*
3½ ounces tempeh
½ tablespoon tamari or soy
   sauce
½ tablespoon maple syrup
½ teaspoon smoked paprika
¼ teaspoon ground cumin
1 tablespoon extra virgin olive oil

**1.** For the tempeh "bacon," slice the tempeh as thinly as you can without it falling apart.

**2.** Combine the rest of the tempeh ingredients except the olive oil in a shallow bowl. Coat the tempeh slices with the marinade on both sides and leave to marinate for 5 minutes.

**3.** Heat the olive oil in a frying pan over high heat

and, when it's hot, add the tempeh and cook for 1–2 minutes on each side until both sides are browned and crisp. Transfer onto a piece of paper towel to cool.

**4.** Toast the slices of bread, if desired. Layer the bottom slice of bread or toast with vegan mayonnaise (if using), followed by slices of avocado, tomato, tempeh "bacon," a little seasoning, and the lettuce leaf. Top with the other slice of bread/toast and serve.

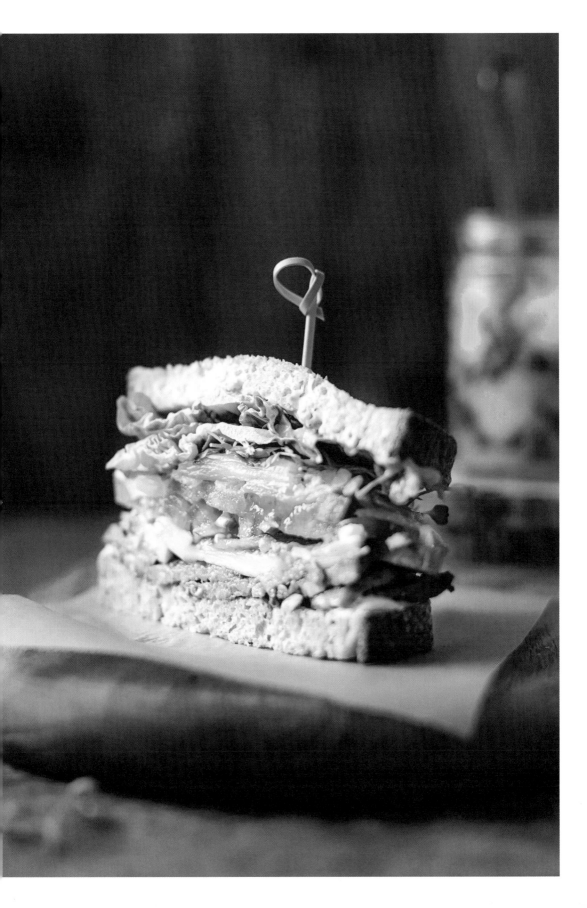

# VERY BERRY PROTEIN SMOOTHIE

SERVES 1 | **Prep time:** 5 minutes

**Nutrition per serving:** 377 cal | 17g protein | 54g carbs | 9g fat | 11.3g fiber

⅔ cup frozen berries

½ banana

1 cup oat milk

¼ cup (1 ounce) oats

1 tablespoon sunflower seed
   protein powder

2 sprigs of fresh mint

**1.** Place all the ingredients except the mint in a blender and blend for 30 seconds until smooth.

**2.** Garnish with the fresh mint sprigs.

# PINA-KALE-ADA PROTEIN SMOOTHIE

SERVES 1 | **Prep time:** 5 minutes

**Nutrition per serving:** 459 cal | 19.3g protein | 52.2g carbs | 17.5g fat | 5.5g fiber

2½ ounces pineapple (fresh,
   frozen, or canned)

½ cup kale (or use cavolo nero
   or spinach)

½ banana

¾ cup coconut water

⅓ cup coconut milk (from a can)

2 tablespoons sunflower seed
   protein powder

**1.** Place all the ingredients in a blender and blend for up to 1 minute until smooth.

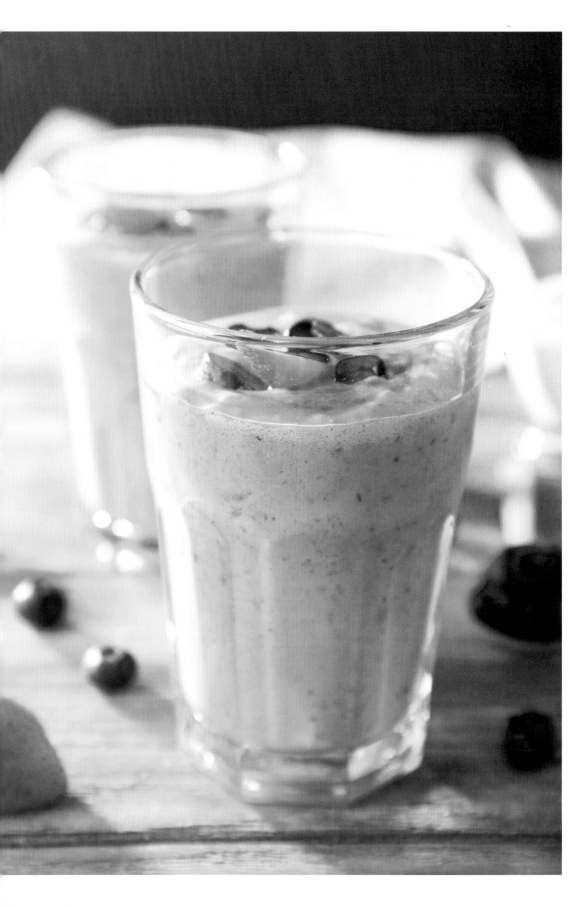

# COCONUT FRENCH TOAST WITH CHERRY COMPOTE

SERVES 1 | **Prep time:** 10 minutes | **Cook time:** 10 minutes
Nutrition per serving: 648 cal | 15.1g protein | 78.6g carbs | 29.7g fat | 8.1g fiber

*Bread often gets a bad rap, but unless you have a gluten intolerance, whole grain and especially sourdough loaves can be a delicious and nutritious base to a meal. Sourdough undergoes a slow, natural fermentation process that gives flavor, enhancing some nutrients and making it easier on the digestive system.*

¼ cup coconut milk (from a can)

1 teaspoon ground cinnamon

1 teaspoon vanilla extract

1 tablespoon almond meal

1 tablespoon gram flour

1 teaspoon maple syrup

pinch of sea salt

1 large or 2 smaller slices of
  sourdough bread (try a rye or
  spelt loaf)

2 teaspoons coconut oil

*For the cherry compote:*

⅔ cup frozen pitted sweet
  cherries

2 tablespoons coconut milk
  (from a can)

1 tablespoon water

**1.** Whisk together the coconut milk, cinnamon, vanilla, almond meal, gram flour, maple syrup, and salt in a large, wide bowl. Place the sourdough slices in the batter and allow to soak for a minute on each side.

**2.** Heat a frying pan and add the coconut oil. Fry the French toast for 2–3 minutes on each side until golden brown.

**3.** Meanwhile, place all the ingredients for the cherry compote in a small saucepan on medium-high heat and simmer for 5 minutes until the cherries are soft and the liquid has thickened.

**4.** Serve the French toast with the cherry compote.

# MUSHROOMS, PINE NUTS, AND ARUGULA ON RYE BREAD

SERVES 1 | **Prep time:** 10 minutes | **Cook time:** 10 minutes
Nutrition per serving: 405 cal | 12.3g protein | 27.4g carbs | 29.5g fat | 7.3g fiber

*German-style rye bread is naturally fermented, dense, dark, chewy, and tangy. It goes beautifully with meaty mushrooms, peppery arugula, and crunchy pine nuts. You could of course substitute another whole grain bread, if preferred.*

¼ cup pine nuts

½ tablespoon olive oil

1 garlic clove, finely chopped

2 portobello mushrooms, finely sliced

1 tablespoon chopped fresh parsley

1 slice of German-style rye bread, toasted

1 cup arugula

sea salt and ground black pepper

**1.** Toast the pine nuts for 1–2 minutes in a dry frying pan until they start to take on some color. Set aside.

**2.** Heat the oil in a saucepan, then sauté the garlic and mushrooms for 5 minutes or until softened. Remove from the heat and stir in the parsley.

**3.** Layer the toasted bread with the arugula and mushroom mix, and top with the toasted pine nuts. Season to taste and serve.

# HUMMUS, AVOCADO, AND TOMATO TOAST

SERVES 1 | Prep time: 5 minutes | Cook time: 2 minutes
Nutrition per serving: 549 cal | 12.7g protein | 49.7g carbs | 33.4g fat | 8.6g fiber

*Hummus is a hugely popular plant-based staple that's available almost everywhere now. Made from a base of garbanzo beans and tahini, it's high in fiber, healthy fats, and plant proteins. It's a superquick solution for adding flavor and substance to any meal, from a salad bowl to a simple slice of toast.*

1 slice of sourdough bread (try spelt or whole grain), toasted

⅓ cup hummus (see below; the remaining hummus will keep in the refrigerator for 2–3 days)

½ avocado, sliced

1 tomato, sliced

sea salt and ground black pepper

*For the hummus:*

1 14-ounce can garbanzo beans, drained and rinsed

1 garlic clove

1 tablespoon tahini

juice of 1 lemon

1 tablespoon extra virgin olive oil

**1.** For the hummus, put the garbanzo beans in a food processor with the garlic, tahini, lemon juice, and oil. Season to taste, then blend for 30 seconds.

**2.** Use a spatula to scrape down the sides of the bowl, then blend for another 30 seconds or until smooth. Check the seasoning and add more lemon juice and a splash of water to loosen, if needed.

**3.** Layer the toasted bread with the hummus, avocado, and tomato slices. Season to taste and serve.

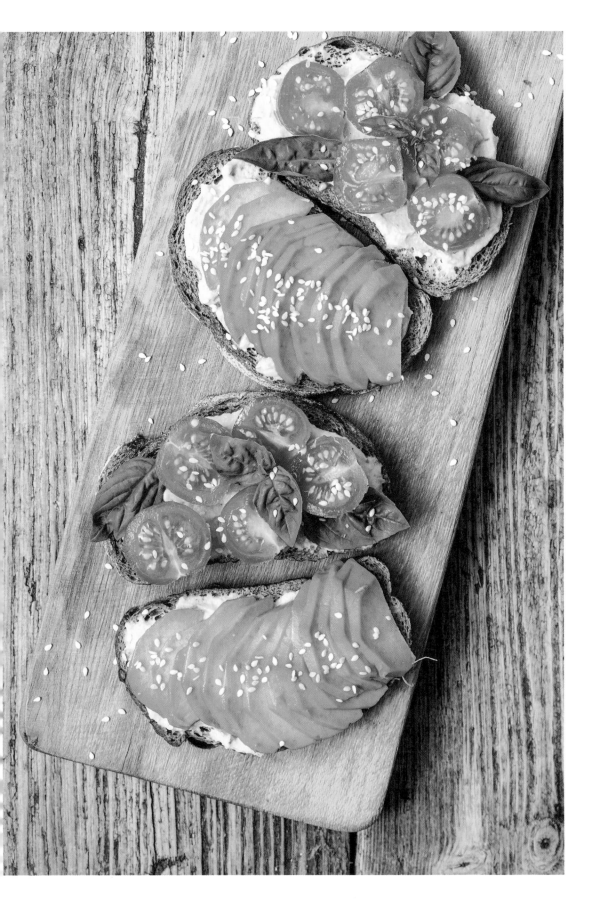

# CORN AND ZUCCHINI FRITTERS WITH SALSA

SERVES 1 | **Prep time:** 10 minutes | **Cook time:** 15 minutes
**Nutrition per serving:** 421 cal | 16.6g protein | 50.9g carbs | 17.3g fat | 10.5g fiber

*These hassle-free fritters cleverly use the vegetables' own moisture to create the batter when combined with the flour. They're perfect for a weekend brunch that everyone will enjoy.*

*For the salsa:*

½ scallion, finely sliced

sea salt and ground black
  pepper

juice of ½ lime

¼ avocado, chopped

1 tomato, chopped

2 tablespoons chopped fresh
  cilantro

1 zucchini

1 scallion, finely sliced

¼ cup corn kernels

1 teaspoon Dijon mustard

½ cup (2 ounces) gram flour

pinch of kala namak (or use
  sea salt)

¼ teaspoon garlic powder

grinding of black pepper

2 tablespoons chopped fresh
  parsley

10 fresh chives, chopped

½ tablespoon olive oil

**1.** For the salsa, place the scallion in a bowl, then season and add the lime juice. Add the avocado, tomato, and cilantro and mix well. Set aside to allow the flavors to combine while you make the fritters.

**2.** Grate the zucchini into a bowl and add all the other fritter ingredients, apart from the olive oil. Mix to combine, then leave for 5 minutes or so to allow the gram flour to absorb the moisture from the zucchini.

**3.** Heat the olive oil in a frying pan. Spoon in five fritters and cook over medium-high heat for 2–3 minutes on each side, until brown on the outside and cooked through in the middle.

**4.** Serve the fritters alongside the salsa.

# CHICKPEA OMELET MUSHROOMS

SERVES 1 | **Prep time:** 10 minutes | **Cook time:** 15 minutes
Nutrition per serving: 533 cal | 23.7g protein | 78.7g carbs | 23.7g fat | 12g fiber

*A hearty and nutritious meal, perfect to share with friends. For the full breakfast experience, serve a slice of sourdough toast and a scant ½ cup of cooked baked beans with the mushrooms and tomatoes.*

2 large portobello mushrooms

8 cherry tomatoes on the vine

kala namak or regular salt and
 black pepper

olive oil

¼ red bell pepper, finely
 chopped

¼ cup (1 ounce) gram flour

¼ cup oat milk

½ tablespoon nutritional yeast

large pinch of ground turmeric

1 teaspoon Dijon mustard

large pinch of garlic powder

large pinch of onion powder

2 tablespoons finely chopped
 fresh chives

2 tablespoons finely chopped
 fresh parsley

**1.** Preheat the oven to 350°F (180°C). Line a baking sheet with parchment paper.

**2.** Cut out the mushroom stems and a little of the insides to make a well in each mushroom cap. Retain the cuttings. Place the hollowed-out mushrooms on the baking sheet with the tomatoes still on the vine. Season and drizzle with 1 tablespoon of olive oil and cook for 20 minutes.

**3.** Meanwhile, finely chop the mushroom stems and insides. Place in a pan with the chopped pepper and a little olive oil and cook over medium-high heat for about 5 minutes or until softened.

**4.** Whisk together the gram flour, milk, nutritional yeast, turmeric, mustard, garlic and onion powders, a pinch of salt, and grind of pepper in a bowl. Add the chopped herbs and the mushroom/pepper mix and combine.

**5.** Remove the mushrooms and tomatoes from the oven. Pour off any liquid inside the mushrooms onto the baking sheet. Divide the batter between the mushrooms, then return to the oven and cook for a further 12–15 minutes until the batter is cooked.

# SCRAMBLED TOFU

SERVES 1 | **Prep time:** 10 minutes | **Cook time:** 15 minutes
**Nutrition per serving:** 304 cal | 19.1g protein | 29.8g carbs | 11.3g fat | 3.6g fiber

*This is a really easy way to cook flavorful tofu, and is a filling breakfast dish. Turmeric is the true superfood spice, supporting liver and antioxidant function, and is a potent anti-inflammatory. Here it gives both taste and color to the dish.*

1 teaspoon olive oil

¼ onion, chopped

¼ cup button mushrooms, chopped

¼ red bell pepper, chopped

3½ ounces firm tofu (organic)

¼ teaspoon ground turmeric

1 teaspoon tamari or soy sauce

1 cup lightly packed fresh parsley, finely chopped

ground black pepper

1 slice of bread (try spelt sourdough or a German-style rye), toasted

**1.** Heat the olive oil in a saucepan and cook the onions, mushrooms, and peppers for 5–10 minutes or until soft.

**2.** Drain the tofu and squeeze out any excess moisture. Crumble the tofu into the onion mixture, add the turmeric and tamari, and mix thoroughly. Cook for 2–3 minutes over medium heat until piping hot.

**3.** Stir the parsley into the tofu and season before serving on the toast.

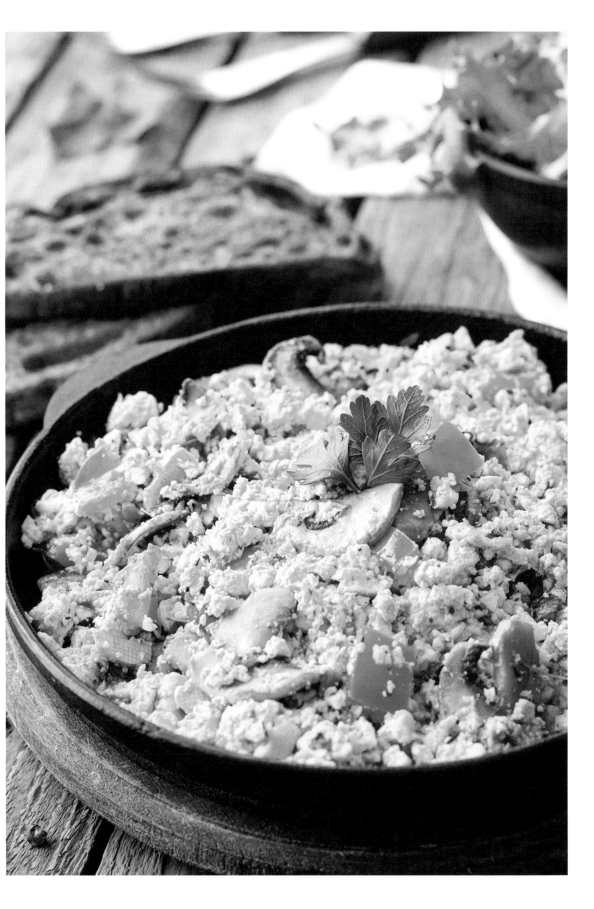

# WALNUT AND BANANA BREAD

SERVES 8 | **Prep time:** 10 minutes | **Cook time:** 1 hour
**Nutrition per 2 slices:** 522 cal | 12.2g protein | 68.5g carbs | 23.3g fat | 7.3g fiber

*Banana bread is great just out of the oven, or you can slice and freeze it, defrosting slices in the toaster for a superquick and convenient breakfast. Enjoy it on its own, or spread with coconut oil, cashew cheese, or a spread of your choice. The addition of sunflower seed protein powder ups the protein content.*

4 tablespoons coconut oil, plus extra for greasing

3–4 very ripe bananas

1⅔ cups (7 ounces) self-rising flour

½ cup (2 ounces) almond meal

3 tablespoons sunflower seed protein powder

1 teaspoon baking powder

⅓ cup (3 ounces) light muscovado sugar

4 dates, finely chopped

4–5 tablespoons oat milk

⅔ cup (3 ounces) walnuts, finely chopped

¼ teaspoon grated nutmeg

½ teaspoon vanilla extract

pinch of sea salt

**1.** Preheat the oven to 350°F (180°C). Brush a loaf pan with a little oil, then line with parchment paper.

**2.** Mash the bananas with the coconut oil in a large mixing bowl. Add all the other ingredients and mix until just combined, but don't overwork the batter.

**3.** Scrape the mixture into the pan. Bake for 1 hour, covering the top with foil if it starts to brown too quickly. The bread is ready when a skewer inserted into the center comes out clean. If it's not ready, return to the oven and cook for a further 10 minutes. Cool for 10 minutes before slicing and serving.

# CRUSHED CREAMY BASIL CHILI PEAS ON TOAST

SERVES 1 | **Prep time:** 10 minutes | **Cook time:** 7 minutes
**Nutrition per serving:** 416 cal | 19.4g protein | 57.6g carbs | 11.3g fat | 5.7g fiber

*This is a fresh, vibrant breakfast, bringing greens to your plate. Peas are a super eco-friendly crop. They actually give back to the soil as they grow, making it rich and fertilized for other plants in the future. They're best bought frozen, as the freezing process locks in the nutrients.*

⅔ cup frozen peas

3½ ounces silken tofu

7 fresh basil leaves, finely
  chopped (fresh mint would
  also work well)

juice of ½ lemon

½ tablespoon olive oil

pinch of chili flakes

sea salt and ground black
  pepper

2 slices of whole wheat
  sourdough, toasted

**1.** Bring a saucepan of water to a boil and cook the peas for 3–4 minutes or until cooked through. Remove from the heat and drain.

**2.** Mash the peas in a bowl with the tofu, basil, lemon juice, olive oil, chili flakes, and salt and pepper to taste.

**3.** Top the toasted bread with the crushed peas.

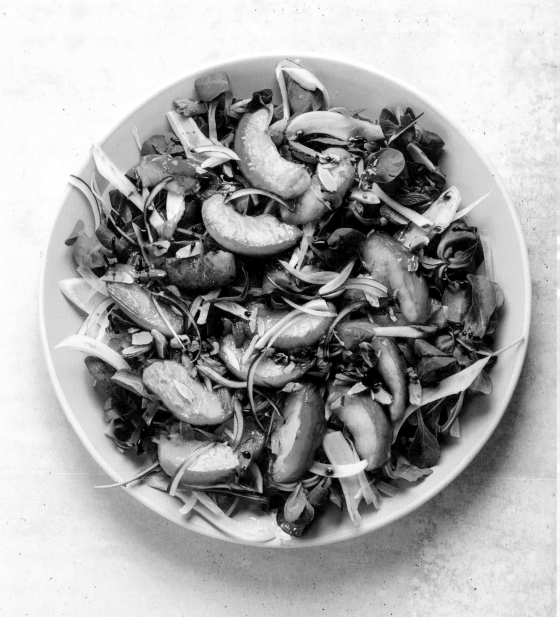

# Soups and Salads

Soups and salads are the backbone of any plant-based diet. They allow you to pack in a load of nutritious foods quickly and easily with minimal prep and hassle—and they're portable, for a meal on the go. There is a seemingly infinite number of ingredient combinations that can be flavored with herbs and spices and made rich with stocks, dressings, and plant oils. You can also add nuts or legumes to create a filling, sustaining dish. Don't be afraid to fill up on a good portion, and make sure you're eating enough, as they're most often nutrient-dense and have a lower calorie count.

*Peaches and spiced garbanzo beans with arugula dressing (page 97)*

# ROASTED CARROT AND LENTIL SALAD

SERVES 1 | **Prep time:** 15 minutes | **Cook time:** 30 minutes
**Nutrition per serving:** 503 cal | 21g protein | 62.3g carbs | 20.2g fat | 18.8g fiber

*This is a classic example of how filling and satisfying plant-based dishes are. It might seem a large portion, but it contains only the calories of an average healthy meal. You can make it in advance and just add the arugula at the last minute (the flavors will marry together beautifully), or serve it warm.*

5 ounces carrots, peeled and chopped

1 tablespoon olive oil, plus 1 teaspoon for roasting

¼ teaspoon garam masala

sea salt and ground black pepper

¼ red onion, finely diced

1½ teaspoons apple cider vinegar

1 14-ounce can green lentils (or use dried, if you prefer; follow the instructions on the package)

1 teaspoon maple syrup

1 tablespoon chopped fresh parsley

1 tablespoon chopped fresh mint

1 cup arugula

**1.** Preheat the oven to 400°F (200°C).

**2.** Toss together the carrots, 1 teaspoon of oil, the garam masala, and a little salt and pepper in a bowl. Spread the mixture on a parchment-lined baking sheet and roast for 30 minutes.

**3.** Meanwhile, place the onion and apple cider vinegar in the same bowl used for the carrots. Leave to marinate while the carrots cook.

**4.** Drain and rinse the lentils.

**5.** Once the carrots are roasted, add them to the bowl of marinating onions along with the lentils and all the remaining ingredients. Toss together to mix well and serve warm or cold. If making in advance, add the arugula just before serving.

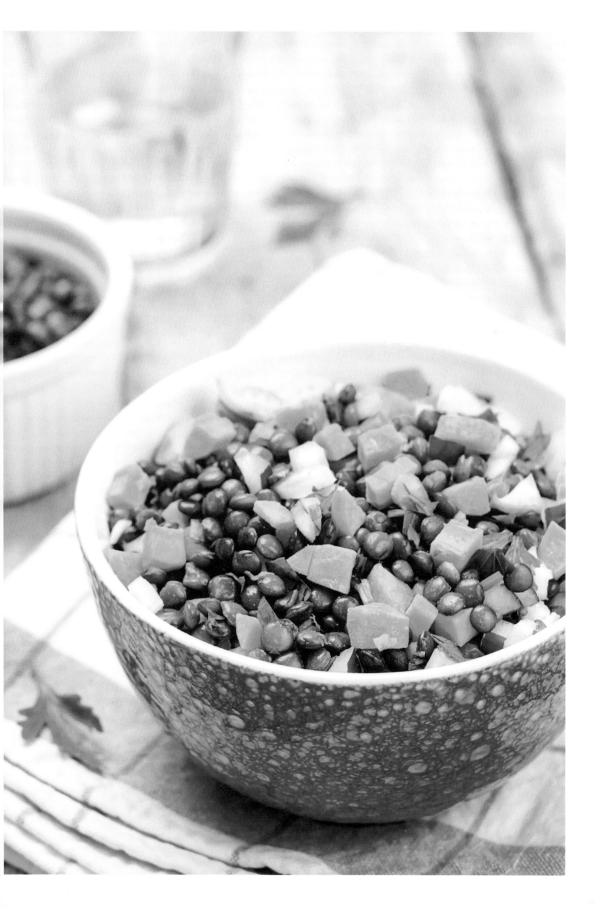

# WATERCRESS, BASIL, AND ALMOND SOUP

SERVES 1 | **Prep time:** 10 minutes | **Cook time:** 10 minutes
**Nutrition per serving:** 428 cal | 18g protein | 22.2g carbs | 33.1g fat | 8.6g fiber

*The advice to "eat your greens" is sometimes easier said than done, but this soup is one of the tastiest and most effective means of achieving it. It's packed full of fragrant, nutritious greens, while the almonds really fill you up and give a delicious, rich creaminess to the soup.*

1 teaspoon olive oil

½ onion, roughly chopped

1 garlic clove, finely chopped

1 cup water, plus more
   if needed

1 teaspoon vegan bouillon
   powder

½ cup (2 ounces) almond meal

2½ cups spinach

1 cup lightly packed fresh basil
   leaves

1½ cups watercress

sea salt and ground black
   pepper

juice of ¼ lemon

**1.** Heat the olive oil in a saucepan over high heat, then add the onion and garlic, splashing the pan with a little water if needed to create steam and keep the onions from sticking. Cook for around 5 minutes or until the onions are soft.

**2.** Add the water, bouillon powder, and almond meal. Bring to a boil, then reduce the heat and add the spinach, basil, and watercress. They will wilt in under a minute. Season with salt, pepper, and the lemon juice.

**3.** Blend the soup with a hand blender until smooth and creamy, or use an upright blender or food processor, but be very careful to seal the container, as the liquid will be very hot.

# PEACHES AND SPICED GARBANZO BEANS WITH ARUGULA DRESSING

SERVES 1 | **Prep time:** 15 minutes | **Cook time:** 30 minutes
**Nutrition per serving:** 643 cal | 21.1g protein | 61.8g carbs | 30.8g fat | 20.5g fiber

*These crispy spiced garbanzo beans are great to add crunch to a salad, or even as a snack on their own. You can play around with different flavors: try garam masala to create an Indian feel, or smoked paprika and lime juice for a Mexican twist. They're full of protein and fiber, so good for filling you up.*

1 14-ounce can garbanzo beans, drained and rinsed

2 tablespoons olive oil

1 tablespoon ras el hanout

sea salt and ground black pepper

1 peach

2 teaspoons apple cider vinegar

1 teaspoon maple syrup

1 cup arugula

**1.** Preheat the oven to 400°F (200°C).

**2.** Combine the garbanzo beans with 1 tablespoon of olive oil, the ras el hanout, and a little salt and pepper in a bowl until all the beans are coated well. Spread out on a parchment-lined baking sheet and bake for 15 minutes, then give the baking sheet a shake before returning to the oven for a further 10 minutes.

**3.** Meanwhile, cut the peach into eight wedges, discarding the pit. In a hot griddle pan or under a hot broiler, sear the peach wedges for 3 minutes on each side.

**4.** Make the vinaigrette by combining the remaining olive oil with the vinegar and maple syrup and season to taste.

**5.** While still warm, toss the peaches, arugula, and garbanzo beans in the vinaigrette and serve.

# BUCKWHEAT NOODLE, SEAWEED, ASPARAGUS, AND EDAMAME SALAD

SERVES 1 | **Prep time:** 10 minutes | **Cook time:** 10 minutes
Nutrition per serving: 454 cal | 21.2g protein | 65.2g carbs | 10.9g fat | 13.3g fiber

*Soba noodles are traditionally made from buckwheat, which is a completely gluten-free, high-protein grain, and has no relation to wheat at all. The noodles have a tendency to be a bit sticky, so it's important to stir them well after adding them to the pan, and to rinse them afterward.*

¼ cucumber

1 sheet nori

juice of 1 lime

3 ounces 100 percent
  buckwheat (soba) noodles

scant ½ cup frozen edamame

1½ ounces thin asparagus

½ tablespoon sesame oil

½ tablespoon tamari or soy
  sauce

2 tablespoons finely chopped
  fresh cilantro

**1.** Slice the cucumber as thinly as you can, then slice the rounds in half and place them in a shallow bowl. Tear the nori sheet into bite-sized pieces and add to the bowl along with the lime juice, and set aside while you prepare the rest of the ingredients.

**2.** Bring a saucepan of water to a boil and add the noodles, stirring well to prevent them from clumping together. Cook for 3 minutes, then add the edamame and asparagus and cook for a further 3 minutes. Drain, then rinse under cold water.

**3.** Add the cold noodles, asparagus, and edamame to the cucumber and nori, along with the sesame oil, tamari, and cilantro. Mix well to combine and serve.

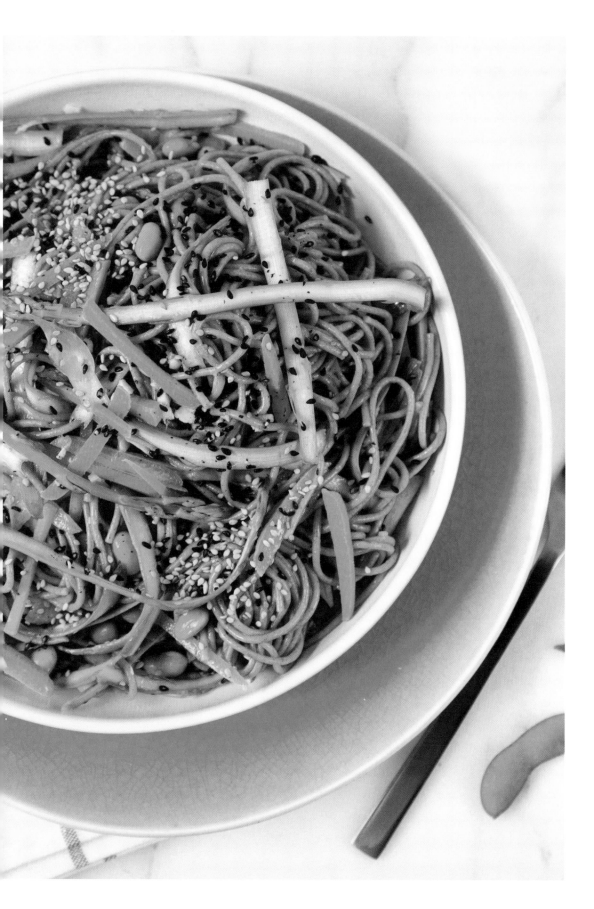

# ROASTED ARTICHOKE, WHITE BEAN, AND TOMATO SALAD

SERVES 1 | **Prep time:** 15 minutes | **Cook time:** 20 minutes
**Nutrition per serving:** 451 cal | 13.9g protein | 37.1g carbs | 28.4g fat | 15.5g fiber

*This is a fresh and vibrant salad, simple to make and able to be prepped ahead of time—in fact, a few hours of the flavors getting to know one another enhances it, so it's perfect in a packed lunch. This recipe uses butter beans, which are large and creamy, but any white bean will do.*

8–10 frozen artichoke hearts (or use 1 14-ounce can artichoke hearts)

2 tablespoons extra virgin olive oil

juice of 1 lemon

sea salt and ground black pepper

1 14-ounce can butter beans

12 cherry tomatoes, halved

¼ onion, finely chopped (optional)

3 tablespoons finely chopped fresh parsley

¾ cup watercress

1. Preheat the oven to 400°F (200°C).

2. If using frozen artichoke hearts, allow them to thaw; if using canned, drain them well, squeezing out all the water. Cut the hearts into quarters, place in a bowl, add half the oil and half the lemon juice, and season with salt and pepper. Pour the mixture onto a parchment-lined baking sheet and place in the oven for 20 minutes, until roasted with slightly charred edges.

3. Meanwhile, use the same mixing bowl to combine the butter beans with the remaining lemon juice and olive oil. Add the tomatoes, onion (if using), and parsley, then season and mix well. Set aside to marinate.

4. Allow the artichokes to cool for a few minutes before adding them to the bean and tomato mixture.

5. When ready to serve, use the watercress leaves as a base and pour the bean, artichoke, and tomato mixture over them.

# VEGAN CAESAR SALAD

SERVES 1 | **Prep time:** 10 minutes
**Nutrition per serving:** 595 cal | 23.3g protein | 43.6g carbs | 38.5g fat | 12.3g fiber

*Traditional Caesar salad, with its high-fat dressing, is probably one of the least healthy salads; this recipe, however, gives it a plant-based makeover, replacing the animal fats with healthy ones from cashews, olive oil, and avocado. It's just as tasty but fills you only with goodness.*

1 head baby gem lettuce, roughly chopped

½ avocado, chopped

juice of ½ lemon

4 tablespoons nutritional yeast

3 tablespoons raw cashew nuts

⅓ garlic clove (or use ¼ teaspoon garlic powder)

½ teaspoon Dijon mustard

1–2 tablespoons water

2 tablespoons oat milk

½ tablespoon olive oil

scant 1 cup croutons

sea salt and ground black pepper

**1.** Place the lettuce and avocado in a bowl.

**2.** Put the lemon juice, yeast, nuts, garlic, mustard, 1 tablespoon of water, oat milk, and oil into a blender and blend for 2–3 minutes, scraping down the sides as necessary, until smooth. Add another tablespoon of water for a looser consistency.

**3.** Pour the dressing over the avocado and lettuce. Scatter the croutons on top, then season, toss, and serve.

# ITALIAN WHITE BEAN AND CAVOLO NERO SOUP

SERVES 2 | **Prep time:** 15 minutes | **Cook time:** 40 minutes
**Nutrition per serving:** 415 cal | 20.2g protein | 66.2g carbs | 5.4g fat | 15.3g fiber

*A simple, hearty soup of classic Italian ingredients and flavors: pasta, beans, tomatoes, and a soffritto base of onion, carrot, and celery sautéed in olive oil. Everything you need to keep you nourished, full, and satisfied.*

½ tablespoon olive oil

½ onion, finely chopped

1 garlic clove, finely chopped

½ carrot, finely chopped

½ celery stick, finely chopped

½ 14-ounce can chopped
tomatoes

2 cups water

2 teaspoons vegan bouillon
powder

1 teaspoon dried oregano

grinding of black pepper

1 14-ounce can white beans
(cannellini, butter, etc.), drained
and rinsed

¼ cup whole wheat pasta

⅔ cup cavolo nero

2 slices whole grain sourdough
bread, toasted

**1.** Place the oil, onion, garlic, carrot, and celery in a large saucepan and sauté over medium heat for 10 minutes; add a splash of water if it starts to stick to the base of the pan.

**2.** Add the tomatoes, water, bouillon, oregano, and black pepper and simmer for 10 minutes.

**3.** Add the beans and pasta and simmer for a further 15 minutes.

**4.** Strip the cavolo nero leaves from their woody stalks and discard the stalks. Rip up the leaves and add to the soup pot, then simmer for 5 minutes.

**5.** Serve a slice of toasted bread with each portion of the soup. You could also add a portion of dairy-free pesto (page 125) for extra indulgence.

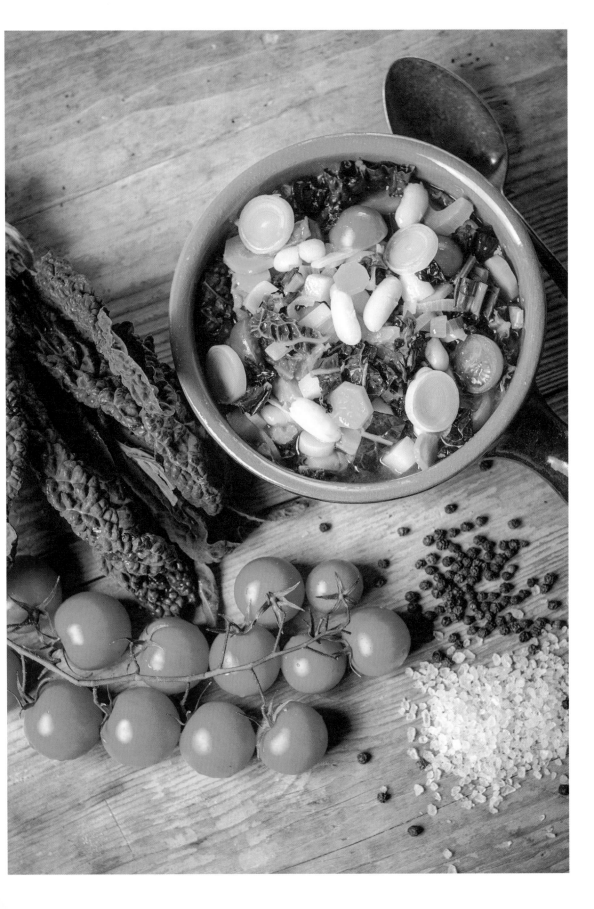

# BUTTERNUT, MACADAMIA, AND SAGE SOUP

SERVES 2 | **Prep time:** 15 minutes | **Cook time:** 45 minutes
**Nutrition per serving:** 471 cal | 10.7g protein | 62.2g carbs | 24.2g fat | 10.1g fiber

*Butternut squash and sage are a classic combination. Roasting the vegetables is such a great way to intensify their flavor, and you can even roast them in advance; then all you have to do is blend everything together when you're ready to create a delicious, satisfying soup in minutes.*

1 pound 1½ ounces butternut squash, diced into ½-inch cubes

½ onion

1 garlic clove

½ tablespoon olive oil

sea salt and ground black pepper

⅓ cup macadamia nuts

2 tablespoons fresh sage leaves

2¾ cups boiling water

1½ teaspoons vegan bouillon powder

2 slices pumpernickel rye bread, toasted

**1.** Preheat the oven to 350°F (180°C).

**2.** Place the squash, onion, and garlic (still in their skins) in a bowl with the olive oil and season with salt and pepper. Toss together to coat before placing on a parchment-lined baking tray. Roast in the oven for 30–40 minutes or until cooked through.

**3.** Peel the garlic clove and onion and add to a large saucepan with the squash and the rest of the ingredients, except the bread. Bring to a boil, then use a hand blender to blend everything together for up to 1 minute or until smooth (you may have to do this in batches).

**4.** Serve a slice of toasted bread with each portion of the soup.

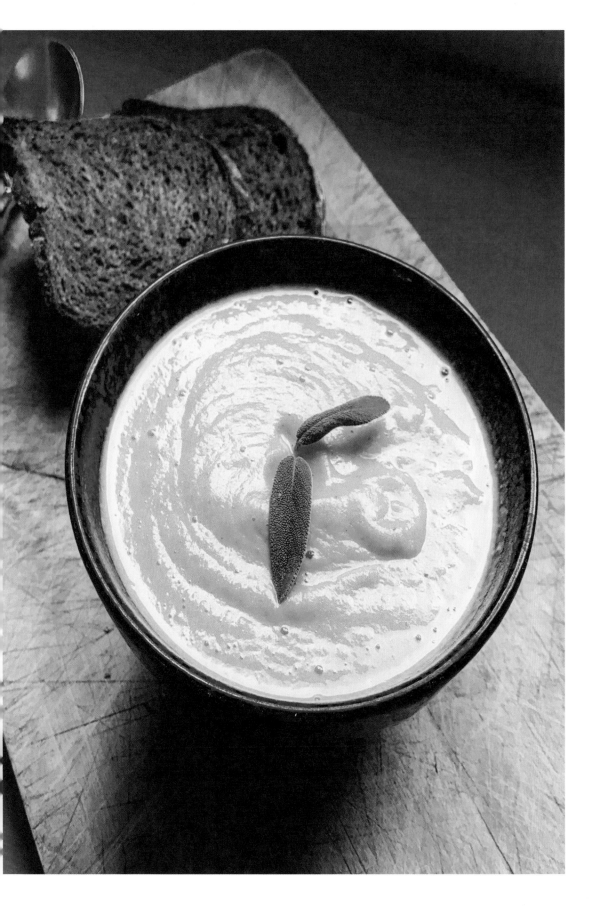

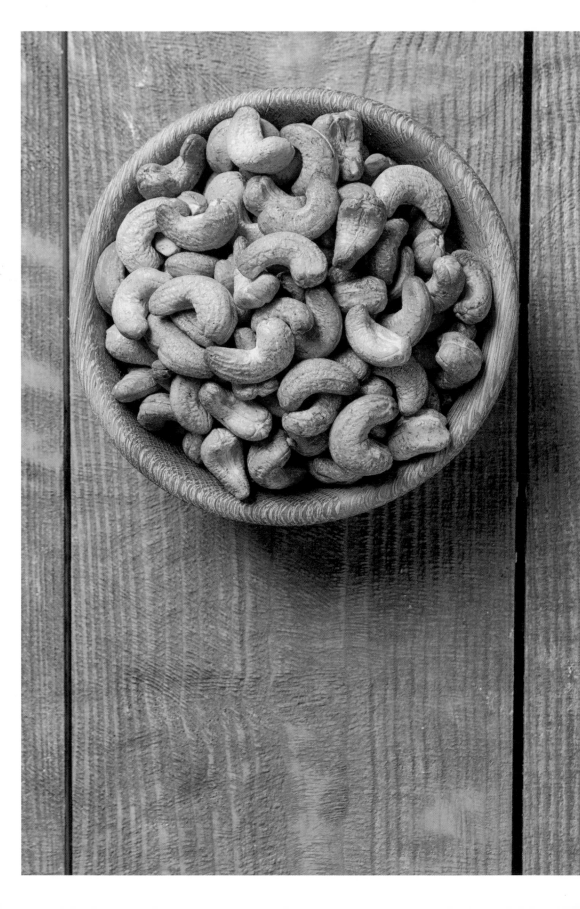

# Mini Meals

---

The way we eat isn't just about biochemistry and sustenance. We have a strong psychological relationship with our diet. The nutritional idea behind "snacks" is that they're small meals that help us with our energy levels when we have a large gap (more than five or six hours) between main meals. Unfortunately, this isn't how snacks are generally registered in our brains. Often we think they "don't count," that they're a bonus, so we tend to eat them on top of what we should be consuming to maintain a healthy weight. Reframing them as smaller or "mini" meals can help with the idea that they're intended purely to satiate hunger and see you through to your next main meal.

*Tamari cashews (page 109)*

# MATCHA POWER BALLS

MAKES 8 BALLS | **Prep time:** 5 minutes
**Nutrition per serving:** 205 cal | 27.7g protein | 15.7g carbs | 15.4g fat | 3.2g fiber

*These are perfect little pick-me-up snack balls to keep you going during the middle part of your eating window. They're packed with healthy fats and proteins from the coconut and almonds, as well as antioxidants and an energy boost from the matcha.*

1 cup (3½ ounces) shredded
  coconut, unsweetened

4 tablespoons almond meal

2 tablespoons maple syrup

1 tablespoon coconut oil

1 tablespoon almond butter

1 teaspoon ground cinnamon

1 teaspoon almond extract

1 tablespoon matcha green tea

**1.** Place all the ingredients in a food processor and blend for 1 minute to form a paste. You may need to stop and scrape the sides of the bowl a few times while blending.

**2.** Shape the mixture into eight balls, around 1 inch in diameter, and enjoy!

# TAMARI CASHEWS

SERVES 4 | **Prep time:** 5 minutes, plus 1–4 hours' marinating | **Cook time:** 20 minutes
**Nutrition per serving:** 171 cal | 5.6g protein | 9.2g carbs | 13.1g fat | 1g fiber

*Nuts are full of healthy fats and protein, ideal to tide you over between main meals. This easy and tasty recipe makes them so addictive that you might end up over-indulging. One great way to prevent this is to eat a piece of fruit alongside the nuts for a complex carb energy boost to help you feel fuller for longer.*

¾ cup raw cashew nuts

1 tablespoon tamari or soy sauce

**1.** Place the cashew nuts and tamari in an airtight container. Give it a shake so the cashews are well coated. Allow to marinate for 1 hour (or up to 4 hours, if desired), giving the container a shake now and again.

**2.** When ready to roast, preheat the oven to 340°F (170°C).

**3.** Place the nuts on a parchment-lined baking sheet and cook for 20 minutes. Remove from the oven and leave to cool and crisp up.

**4.** Divide the nuts into four portions and store three of the portions in an airtight container for up to 2 weeks.

# SUMMER ROLLS WITH SATAY SAUCE

SERVES 1 | **Prep time:** 20 minutes
**Nutrition per serving:** 210 cal | 7.4g protein | 26.5g carbs | 8.6g fat | 3.9g fiber

*This recipe is a fantastic way to package your vegetables in tasty and portable rolls—you can stuff your rice paper with any vegetables you like. Don't let the rice paper soak for too long, however, or it will become mushy.*

*For the satay sauce:*

1 tablespoon crunchy peanut
  butter

1 teaspoon tamari or soy sauce

½ tablespoon coconut milk (from
  a can)

¼ teaspoon maple syrup

¼ teaspoon garam masala

¼ teaspoon dried chili flakes

juice of ½ lime

*For the summer rolls:*

1 scallion

½ medium carrot

5 sugar snap peas (or use
  bean sprouts)

2-inch piece of cucumber

2 sheets rice paper

6 fresh mint leaves

**1.** Mix all the satay sauce ingredients in a bowl and set aside.

**2.** Cut all the vegetables into fine matchsticks.

**3.** Pour some boiling water into a shallow bowl. Soak a sheet of rice paper for 10 seconds until it starts to soften, then place on a clean dish towel. In the center of the sheet, place 3 mint leaves, then half the cilantro and matchstick vegetables. Fold the bottom of the rice paper up and over the vegetables, then fold the sides in to make an "open envelope" shape. Then roll from the bottom to make a sausage shape; the rice paper will seal itself. Repeat with the second sheet.

**4.** Serve with the satay dipping sauce.

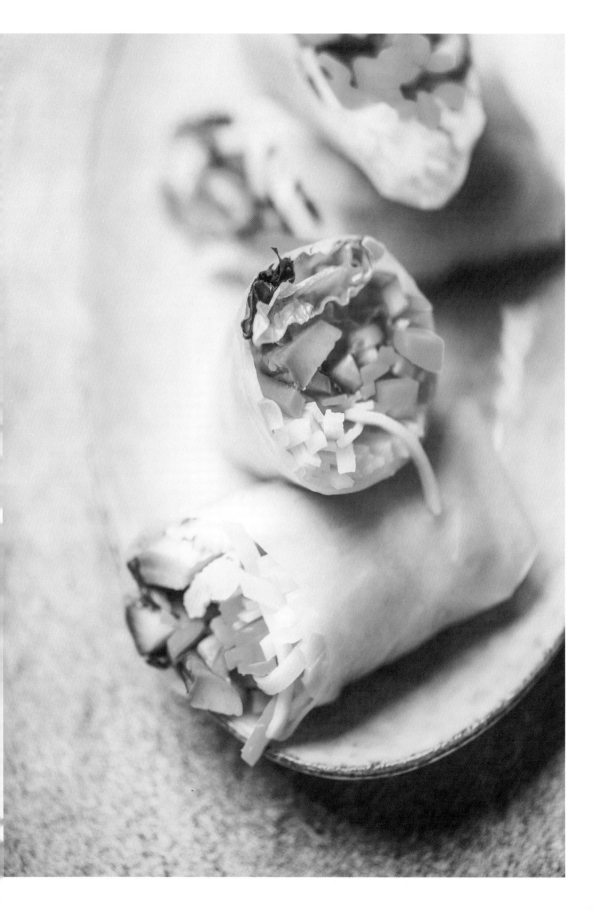

# WALNUT AND MUSHROOM PÂTÉ

SERVES 2 | **Prep time:** 15 minutes, plus 2 hours' refrigeration | **Cook time:** 15 minutes

**Nutrition per serving:** 196 cal | 6.4g protein | 11.2g carbs | 14.9g fat | 2.3g fiber

*This is a wonderful recipe that creates a rich and creamy pâté with only the power of plants. It's great for a mini meal, but can also be used on toast or with salad for a quick supper, or to create delicious canapés. Any leftover pâté can be kept in the fridge for four to five days.*

⅓ cup walnuts, roughly chopped

⅓ cup water

1 tablespoon cornstarch

1½ tablespoons nutritional yeast

1 tablespoon lemon juice

½ tablespoon olive oil

1 tablespoon tamari or soy sauce

¼ teaspoon miso paste

large pinch of garlic powder

large pinch of onion powder

large pinch of smoked paprika

¼ teaspoon dried oregano

ground black pepper

2 button mushrooms

½ cucumber for serving

**1.** Place all the ingredients apart from the mushrooms and cucumbers in a blender and blend for 30 seconds or until smooth. Pour the pâté mixture into a saucepan.

**2.** Add the mushrooms to the blender and pulse for a couple of seconds to chop finely, then add to the pan. Heat the mixture, stirring constantly, for 15 minutes, or until it has thickened.

**3.** Pour the mixture into a flat container and leave in the refrigerator for 2 hours to set.

**4.** Cut the cucumber into 2-inch lengths and serve alongside a portion of the pâté for dipping.

# MUHAMMARA WITH CRUDITÉS (BELL PEPPER AND WALNUT DIP)

SERVES 4 | **Prep time:** 20 minutes | **Cook time:** 20 minutes
**Nutrition per serving:** 246 cal | 5.5g protein | 19.4g carbs | 17.9g fat | 6.4g fiber

*Walnuts are one of the best plant-based sources of omega 3, an anti-inflammatory fatty acid that's great for glowing skin and mood health. Hummus is already a staple of the plant-based diet, and this dip is its little-known cousin. Once you try it, I guarantee it will become a firm favorite, too.*

2 red bell or Romano peppers

⅔ cup walnuts

1 slice of whole grain bread

1 garlic clove

juice of ½ lemon

1 tablespoon pomegranate molasses (or use maple syrup and a little more lemon juice)

1½ teaspoons smoked paprika

¼–½ red chile (depending on how hot you like it)

½ teaspoon garam masala

1½ tablespoons extra virgin olive oil, plus a little extra for roasting the peppers

sea salt and ground black pepper, to taste

2 celery sticks for serving

**1.** Preheat the oven to 450°F (230°C). Rub the peppers in olive oil and place on a baking sheet in the oven for 20 minutes or until the skins start to bubble and blister. Remove from the oven and leave to cool.

**2.** Meanwhile, toast the walnuts in a dry frying pan for 5 minutes.

**3.** Peel and deseed the peppers.

**4.** Place the slice of bread in a food processor or blender and pulse to form bread crumbs. Add the rest of the ingredients, including the pepper flesh and toasted walnuts, and blend until smooth.

**5.** Wash, trim, and cut the celery sticks into 2-inch lengths and serve alongside a portion of the muhammara for dipping. Freeze the remaining portions for later use.

# CHERRY ALMOND CHIA BOWL

SERVES 1 | **Prep time:** 5 minutes, plus 2 hours (or overnight) soaking

**Nutrition per serving:** 220 cal | 7.4g protein | 24.9g carbs | 10.8g fat | 7.9g fiber

*Chia bowls are simple to make and a great way to include chia seeds in your diet, with their healthy omega-3 fatty acids and soluble fiber prebiotics for healthy gut flora. Cherry and almond is a classic combination, but you can try all sorts of flavors. Another favorite is passion fruit and coconut, or cacao and banana.*

1½ tablespoons almond meal

scant ½ cup oat or almond milk

⅓ cup frozen pitted sweet
  cherries

1 tablespoon chia seeds

**1.** Blend the almond meal, milk, and cherries together in a blender for up to 1 minute until smooth.

**2.** Put the chia seeds in a jar or glass, then pour the almond and cherry mixture over them and combine well; if using a jar with a lid, you can give it a good shake.

**3.** Place in the refrigerator for at least 2 hours or overnight.

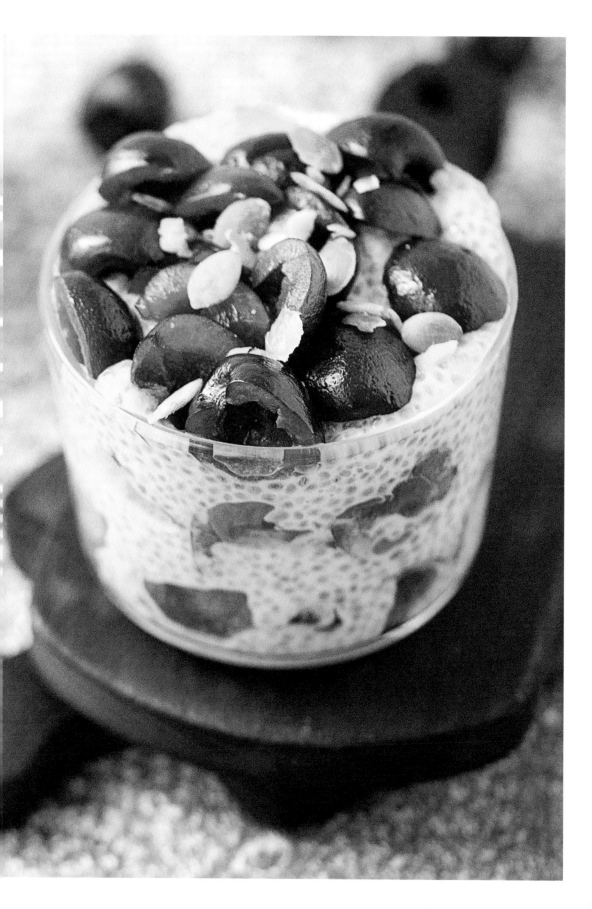

# APPLE CINNAMON CHIPS WITH PEANUT BUTTER

SERVES 1 | **Prep time:** 10 minutes | **Cook time:** 2–3 hours
Nutrition per serving: 190 cal | 5g protein | 29g carbs | 7g fat | 7g fiber

*Apples are high in soluble fiber, so are great for your digestive health. Cinnamon is an insulin mimicker that can help to balance your blood sugar, while peanut butter is a classic snack-time treat, high in healthy fats—but avoid brands with added palm oil or sugar.*

1 apple

1 teaspoon ground cinnamon

1 tablespoon peanut butter

**1.** Preheat the oven to 175°F (80°C). Line a baking sheet with parchment paper.

**2.** Using a sharp knife or mandoline, slice the apple thinly, discarding the seeds. Arrange the apple slices on the baking sheet without overlapping. Sprinkle the cinnamon over the slices.

**3.** Cook for around 1 hour, then flip the slices over and continue cooking for 1–2 hours, flipping occasionally, until the apple slices are no longer moist. Alternatively, use a dehydrator to dry the apple slices, if you have one.

**4.** Serve with peanut butter on top.

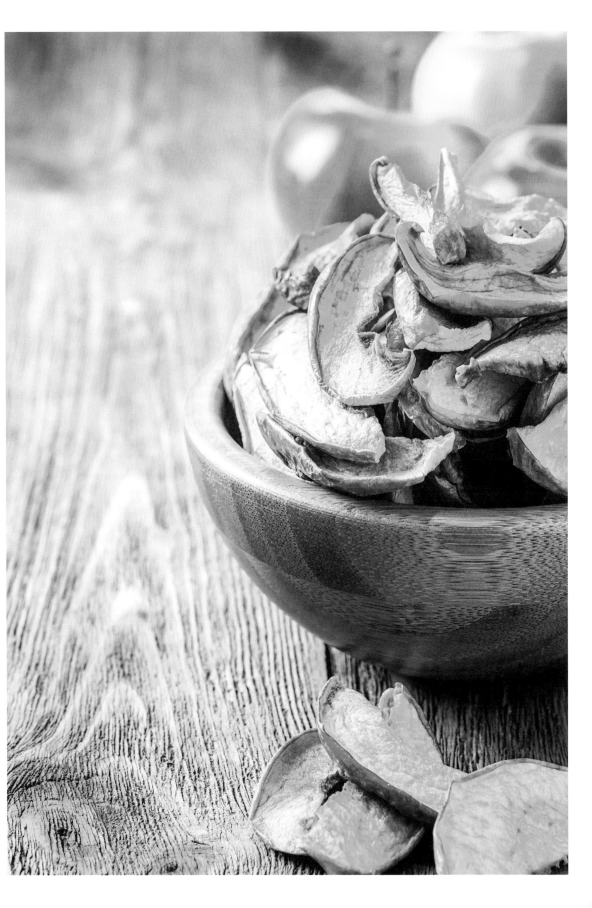

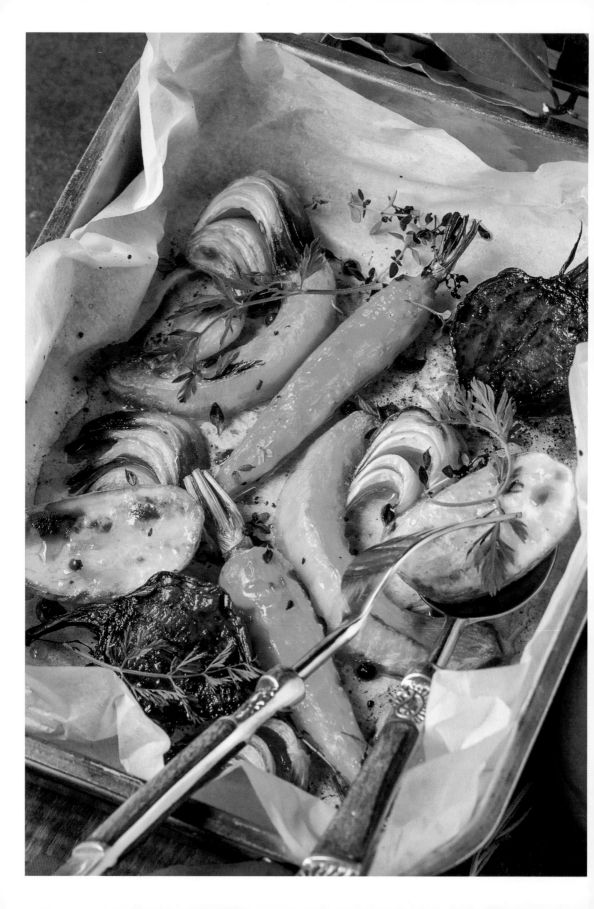

# Main Dishes

---

For many of us, dinner is the main meal of the day, when we tend to have more time to sit down, eat, and talk with others. Following a fasting plan shouldn't change that. In addition, the idea that dishes need to have animal-origin foods in them to be filling and delicious is a total myth. The recipes in this section make dishes that are fragrant, tasty, and satisfying, perfect for sharing with friends and family at the end of a busy day.

*Olive, Herb, and Lemon Vegetable Casserole (page 124)*

# BUTTERNUT LAKSA BOWL

SERVES 2 | **Prep time:** 20 minutes | **Cook time:** 15 minutes
**Nutrition per serving:** 698 cal | 13.7g protein | 47.6g carbs | 47.1g fat | 10.4g fiber

10 ounces butternut squash

1 14-ounce can coconut milk

1¾ cups water

2 star anise

3 tablespoons tamari or soy
   sauce

juice of ½ lime

1 red chile, finely sliced

⅔ cup frozen edamame

½ cup sugar snap peas

1 cup bean sprouts

1 scallion, finely sliced

2 tablespoons chopped fresh
   cilantro

*For the laksa paste:*

½ teaspoon each coriander
   seeds, ground cumin, turmeric

1 green chile

1 large garlic clove

3 tablespoons fresh ginger

3 tablespoons fresh galangal (or
   from a jar)

1 lemongrass stalk

1 cup fresh cilantro

4 lime leaves

1 tablespoon coconut oil

1 tablespoon tamari or soy
   sauce

3 tablespoons water

**1.** Use a spiralizer to create butternut squash noodles; if you don't have a spiralizer, use a vegetable peeler to make ribbons. Set aside.

**2.** To make the laksa paste, place all the ingredients in a food processor and blend for 30 seconds or until smooth.

**3.** Place the laksa paste in a saucepan and cook on high for 5 minutes, stirring continuously so it doesn't stick to the pan or brown too much.

**4.** Add the coconut milk, water, star anise, tamari, lime juice, half the sliced chile, and butternut noodles, and stir well to combine with the cooked paste. Bring to a boil, then reduce the heat and simmer for 5 minutes.

**5.** Add the edamame and sugar snap peas, return to a boil, and then simmer for 2 minutes.

**6.** Ladle the noodles and laksa broth into two bowls. Top each bowl with bean sprouts, scallions, the remaining red chile, and the cilantro.

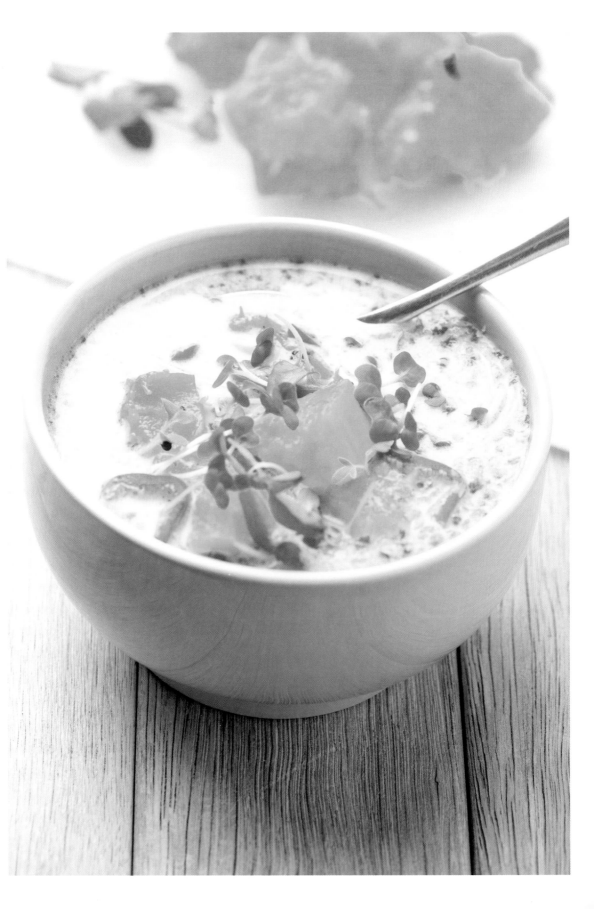

# SWEET POTATO AND SPINACH DAL

SERVES 2 | **Prep time:** 10 minutes | **Cook time:** 45 minutes
**Nutrition per serving:** 428 cal | 18.2g protein | 56.7g carbs | 11.9g fat | 23.1g fiber

*The Indian diet is largely plant-based, so it makes perfect sense that they have delicious, highly spiced vegan staples such as dal. This recipe uses red lentils, because they're readily available and quick and easy to cook. Poppadums are also made from gram flour, meaning they're high in fiber and protein.*

1 cup dried red lentils

1 onion, diced

½ tablespoon coconut oil

3 garlic cloves, finely chopped

1¼-inch piece fresh ginger, finely
  chopped

1–2 chiles (depending on how
  hot you like it), finely chopped

3 teaspoons garam masala

1 teaspoon ground turmeric

10 ounces sweet potatoes,
  diced

scant 3 cups water

2 teaspoons vegan bouillon
  powder

sea salt and ground black
  pepper

juice of ½ lemon

3 tablespoons finely chopped
  fresh cilantro

1 cup spinach

1 tablespoon (dairy-free) coconut
  yogurt

2 store-bought poppadums per
  person

**1.** Rinse the lentils in a sieve and set aside to drain.

**2.** Place the onion and the coconut oil in a large saucepan over medium-low heat for 5 minutes or until starting to soften. Add the garlic, ginger, chiles, garam masala, and turmeric. Cook for a further 5 minutes, stirring to prevent sticking; you can also add a splash of water to help, if needed.

**3.** Add the sweet potatoes along with the drained lentils, water, and bouillon powder; bring to a simmer and cook for 30 minutes, stirring at intervals to prevent it from sticking to the base of the pan.

**4.** Season, then add the lemon juice and cilantro and stir in the spinach for a minute or so until it has wilted.

**5.** Serve with a dollop of coconut yogurt and the poppadums.

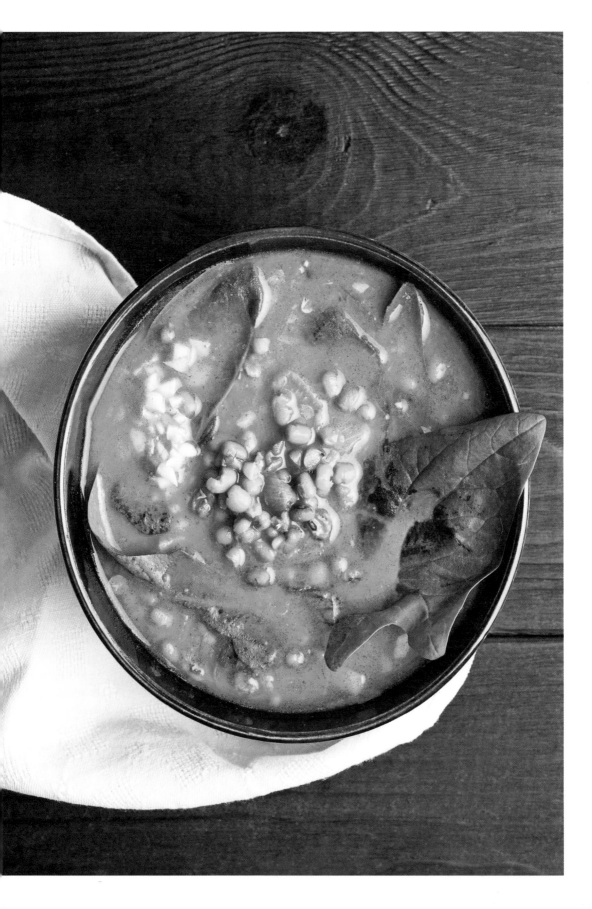

# OLIVE, HERB, AND LEMON VEGETABLE CASSEROLE

SERVES 2 | **Prep time:** 20 minutes | **Cook time:** 40 minutes
Nutrition per serving: 572 cal | 16.1g protein | 56g carbs | 31g fat | 15.4g fiber

*This is a great dish to serve for friends and family. The wonderful colors of the vegetables and the herby olive and lemon dressing will transport you and your guests to a Greek island. It's so easy to cook, but so effective, and you can use whatever vegetables you have in your refrigerator.*

1 sweet potato, chopped

2 green or red bell peppers, chopped

1 onion, chopped into 8 wedges

1 zucchini, chopped

1 carrot, chopped

1 14-ounce can garbanzo beans, drained

3 tablespoons olive oil

juice of 2 lemons

sea salt and ground black pepper

3½ ounces thin asparagus

¾ cup pitted green olives, finely chopped

1 cup lightly packed fresh mint leaves, finely chopped

1 cup lightly packed fresh parsley leaves, finely chopped

**1.** Preheat the oven to 350°F (180°C).

**2.** Place the sweet potatoes, peppers, onions, zucchini, carrots, and garbanzo beans in a bowl, add 1 tablespoon of olive oil, half the lemon juice, and some salt and pepper, and mix to coat everything well. Spread the mixture on a parchment-lined roasting pan and roast in the oven for 30 minutes.

**3.** After 30 minutes, add the asparagus. Give the vegetables and beans a stir, turning if necessary. Return to the oven for a further 10 minutes.

**4.** Meanwhile, make the dressing. Place the olives, mint, and parsley in a bowl or jar. Add the remaining olive oil and lemon juice and season.

**5.** Once the vegetables and beans have finished roasting, remove from the oven, spoon over the dressing, and serve in the pan.

# QUICK PITA "PIZZA" WITH HOMEMADE PESTO

SERVES 2 | **Prep time:** 10 minutes | **Cook time:** 15 minutes
**Nutrition per serving (2 pitas):** 628 cal | 16.8g protein | 61.8g carbs | 32.5g fat | 12.9g fiber

*It's important to have some quick-fix pantry recipes in your repertoire. This one is super simple, and you can use store-bought pesto if you need to make it even quicker. Otherwise, make the pesto in batches and freeze the extra so you have it fresh whenever you need to add a bit of oomph to a dish.*

*Pesto (for 6 pitas):*

2 cups lightly packed fresh basil
  leaves

1 tablespoon walnuts

2 tablespoons pine nuts

1 garlic clove

juice of ½ lemon

3 tablespoons extra virgin
  olive oil

sea salt and ground black
  pepper, to taste

*For the pizzas:*

2 whole grain pitas

2 tablespoons tomato sauce

2 tablespoons antipasti peppers

2 tablespoons antipasti
  artichokes

*For the arugula salad:*

1 cup arugula

¼ tablespoon balsamic vinegar

½ tablespoon olive oil

**1.** Place all the pesto ingredients in a food processor or blender and pulse for 10 seconds.

**2.** Preheat the oven to 400°F (200°C).

**3.** Spread a tablespoon of tomato sauce on each pita. Top each one with a tablespoon of antipasti peppers and artichokes, and drizzle with the pesto. Place in the oven and bake for 15 minutes.

**4.** Toss the arugula leaves in the balsamic vinegar and olive oil, then serve alongside the pizzas.

# BEET BURGER

SERVES 1 | **Prep time:** 20 minutes | **Cook time:** 1 hour 30 minutes
Nutrition per serving: 471 cal | 28.4g protein | 59.7g carbs | 14.1g fat | 13.6g fiber

*Just because you're plant-based doesn't mean you can't enjoy an amazing burger—and these are full of flavor, protein, and vibrancy. You can double up on the patty mixture and freeze the unbaked patties, then cook from frozen for 40 minutes for an easy meal.*

5 ounces beets

2 garlic cloves, unpeeled

½ red onion, unpeeled

4½ ounces firm tofu (organic)

1 tablespoon chia seeds

2 tablespoons nutritional yeast

½ tablespoon tamari or soy
  sauce

2 tablespoons gram flour

1½ teaspoons smoked paprika

1 teaspoon sea salt

ground black pepper

1 whole grain burger bun

½ tablespoon vegan mayonnaise

½ teaspoon mustard

½ tomato, sliced

½ pickle, sliced

1 baby gem lettuce leaf

**1.** Preheat the oven to 350°F (180°C).

**2.** Trim the leaves off the beets, then wrap the beets and garlic in foil. Wrap the red onion in foil separately. Roast for 1 hour, then remove and allow to cool.

**3.** Increase the oven heat to 400°F (200°C). Drain and squeeze out the water from the tofu, then place in a bowl. Finely chop the flesh of the roasted onions and garlic (discard the skins), then add to the bowl. Peel the beets and grate into the bowl.

**4.** Add the chia seeds, nutritional yeast, tamari or soy sauce, gram flour, smoked paprika, salt, and a good grinding of black pepper, and thoroughly combine until the tofu is completely mixed in. The mixture can be firmed up in the refrigerator, if necessary. Create two burger-shaped patties, place on a lined and greased baking sheet, and bake for 30 minutes.

**5.** Meanwhile, prepare your burger bun. Spread mayonnaise and mustard on the bottom half of the bun, then add slices of tomato and pickle. Add the beet patty straight from the oven and top with a lettuce leaf and the top of the bun.

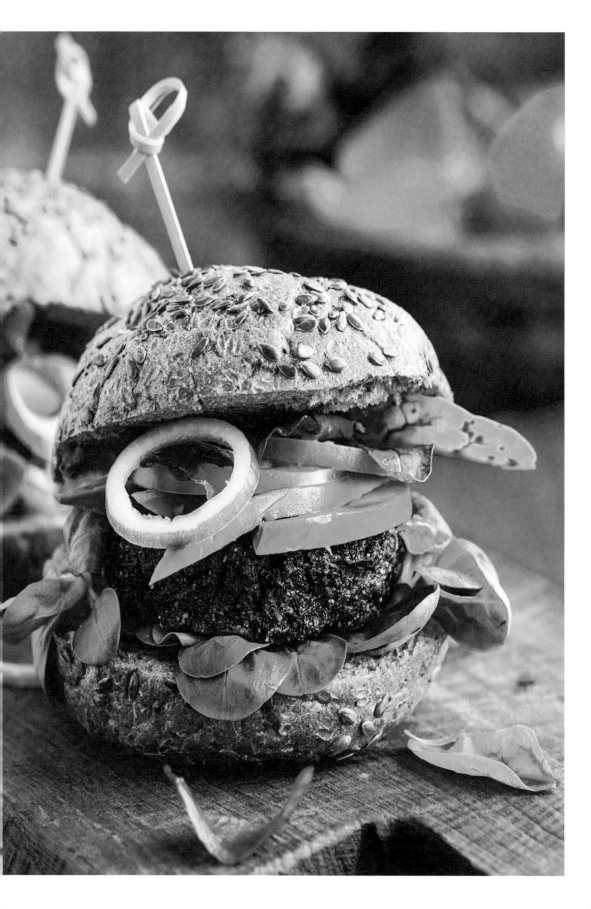

# EGGPLANT WITH MISO TAHINI GLAZE AND SESAME CUCUMBER

---

**SERVES 2**

**Prep time:** 20 minutes, plus 1 hour to press the eggplant (optional) | **Cook time:** 40 minutes

**Nutrition per serving:** 427 cal | 10.3g protein | 33.9g carbs | 26.4g fat | 8.2g fiber

---

2 eggplants

1 tablespoon olive or canola oil

3 tablespoons sweet white miso

2 tablespoons tahini

1 tablespoon sesame oil

1 teaspoon tamari or soy sauce

1 tablespoon pomegranate molasses (or use 1 tablespoon maple syrup and juice of ½ lemon)

*For the sesame cucumber:*

1 cucumber

2 tablespoons brown rice vinegar

1 tablespoon sesame oil

2 teaspoons maple syrup

1 teaspoon sesame seeds

**1.** Cut the eggplant into ½-inch thick slices. If you have time, place them between layers of paper towel and weigh down with books or a heavy cutting board for 1 hour. This will help the eggplant crisp up in the oven.

**2.** Preheat the oven to 400°F (200°C). Place the eggplant slices on a parchment-lined baking sheet, then lightly cover both sides of each round with the oil, using a pastry brush or your fingers. Bake in the oven for 20 minutes.

**3.** Combine the miso, tahini, sesame oil, tamari, and pomegranate molasses in a bowl. Remove the eggplant from the oven, spread half the glaze over one side of the slices (about ½ teaspoon per slice), then return to the oven for 10 minutes. Remove from the oven again, flip the slices over and glaze the other sides with the rest of the miso tahini mixture. Increase the oven temperature to 425°F (220°C) and cook for a final 10 minutes.

**4.** To make the sesame cucumber, while the eggplant is cooking, spiralize the cucumber into wide ribbons, or use a peeler to make long, wide, thin slices. Place in a bowl, add all the other ingredients, and mix well. Leave to marinate while the eggplant cooks.

**5.** When the eggplant is ready, serve on a bed of sesame cucumber.

# SPECIAL FRIED CAULIFLOWER AND QUINOA "RICE"

SERVES 2 | Prep time: 10 minutes | Cook time: 6 minutes
Nutrition per serving: 487 cal | 21g protein | 59g carbs | 18.4g fat | 9.2g fiber

*This is a perfect example of how to make a fresh, vibrant plant-based dish in a matter of minutes. The quinoa can be made ahead of time or bought precooked.*

½ head of cauliflower

1 tablespoon coconut oil

2 scallions, sliced

1 garlic clove, finely chopped

1 red chile, finely chopped

1-inch piece fresh ginger, finely chopped

4½ ounces shiitake mushrooms, sliced

1⅓ cups cooked quinoa

2½ tablespoons tamari or soy sauce

1 head of bok choy, sliced

⅔ cup frozen edamame

3 tablespoons chopped fresh cilantro

juice of ½ lime

*To garnish:*

1 tablespoon chopped fresh cilantro

2 tablespoons bean sprouts

1 tablespoon peanuts, crushed

**1.** Grate the cauliflower to make the "rice" and set aside.

**2.** In a frying pan or wok, heat the coconut oil. Stir-fry the scallions, garlic, chile, ginger, mushrooms, quinoa, and cauliflower "rice" for 3–4 minutes, gradually adding the tamari. If it starts to stick to the base of the pan, add small splashes of water to create steam.

**3.** Finally, add the bok choy, edamame, cilantro, and lime juice, frying for a further minute. Serve with a garnish of chopped cilantro, bean sprouts, and crushed peanuts.

# MEXICAN BLACK BEANS WITH GUACAMOLE

SERVES 2 | Prep time: 15 minutes | Cook time: 40 minutes
Nutrition per serving: 417 cal | 17g protein | 52.3g carbs | 16.5g fat | 22g fiber

½ tablespoon olive oil

1 red onion, diced (save ⅛ for the guacamole)

2 garlic cloves, finely chopped

3 bell peppers (any color), cut into 1-inch dice

½ teaspoon garam masala

1 teaspoon smoked paprika

½ teaspoon chili flakes

1 14-ounce can black beans, drained

1 14-ounce can chopped tomatoes

¾ cup water

1 teaspoon vegan bouillon powder

juice of ½ lime

⅔ cup frozen corn kernels

3 tablespoons fresh cilantro, chopped

salt and ground black pepper

*For the guacamole:*

⅛ red onion (from the stew)

½ tomato, chopped

¼ teaspoon chili flakes

2 teaspoons fresh cilantro

1 ripe avocado

juice of ½ lime

**1.** Heat the olive oil in a saucepan and cook the onion for 5 minutes. Add the garlic and peppers with the spices and cook for a couple more minutes. Add the black beans, tomatoes, water, and bouillon powder. Bring to a simmer and cook with the lid off for 10 minutes, then cover and simmer for a further 20 minutes, stirring occasionally.

**2.** Meanwhile, prepare the guacamole. Finely dice the onion, then place in a bowl with the tomatoes, chili flakes, and cilantro. Mash the avocado with a fork, then add to the bowl with the lime juice and mix well.

**3.** Add the lime juice, corn, and cilantro to the beans, season, and then serve either with sliced avocado or with guacamole.

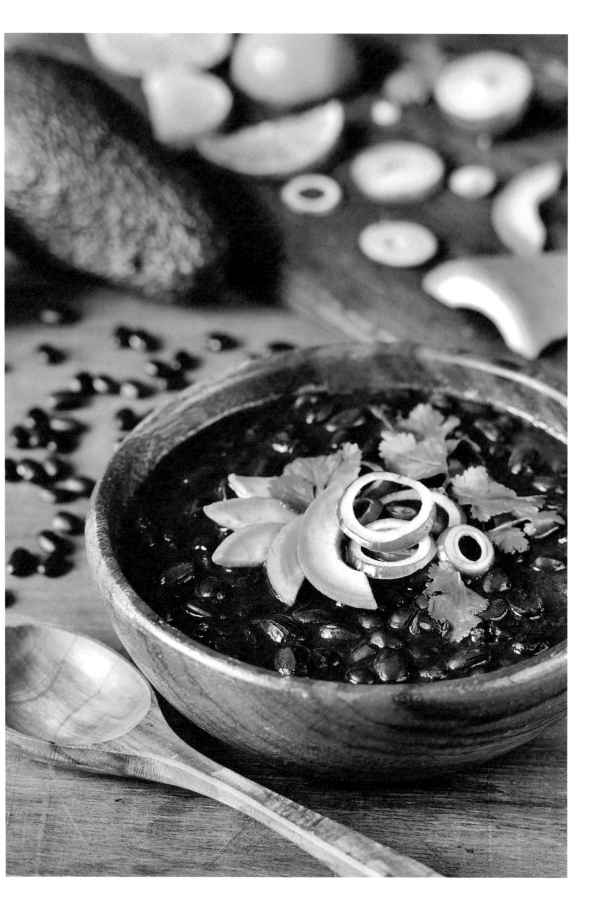

# VEGAN RAGU

SERVES 2 | **Prep time:** 15 minutes | **Cook time:** 1 hour

**Nutrition per serving:** 518 cal | 20.2g protein | 84g carbs | 7.2g fat | 14.9g fiber

*One of the hurdles of moving to a plant-based diet is the thought that you'll miss out on your favorite meat dishes. Pasta with a rich ragu sauce is definitely one of those—however, the vegetable base of most dishes plays a huge part in creating those familiar flavors, and they really do taste just as good.*

½ onion, finely diced

½ carrot, finely diced

½ celery stick, finely diced

¾ cup button mushrooms, finely diced

½ tablespoon olive oil

1 teaspoon dried oregano

2 cups tomato sauce

½ mushroom stock cube or ½ teaspoon vegan bouillon powder

¼ cup red wine

1½ cups Puy lentils (from a can), drained and rinsed

sea salt and ground black pepper

7 ounces whole wheat spaghetti

**1.** Cook the vegetables in the olive oil in a medium pan for 5 minutes. Add the oregano, tomato sauce, stock cube or bouillon, and red wine and bring to a boil. Reduce the heat and simmer, covered, for 50 minutes, stirring occasionally.

**2.** Add the lentils and season, then cook for a further 5 minutes.

**3.** Meanwhile, boil a large pan of water, adding plenty of salt. Cook the spaghetti as per the package instructions to al dente, usually 8–10 minutes. Before draining, set aside a cup of the pasta water.

**4.** Add the drained pasta to the ragu, with a splash of the reserved pasta water. Over a high heat, stirring constantly, coat the spaghetti with the ragu for 2–3 minutes or until the extra water has evaporated. Season with black pepper, if needed, and serve.

# FENNEL, LEEK, AND PEA BAKED BARLEY

SERVES 2 | **Prep time:** 10 minutes | **Cook time:** 50 minutes
**Nutrition per serving:** 536 cal | 19.5g protein | 106g carbs | 3.2g fat | 25g fiber

*Packed with lovely, flavorsome, vibrant spring veggies, this dish is a hassle-free, one-pot wonder. It's baked in the oven, but still feels fresh and light. It gives a good size portion per person because it's so plant-food dense.*

¾ cup pearl barley, washed

2 fennel bulbs, halved, woody stem cut out, and finely sliced

½ cup new potatoes, quartered

1 leek, cut into ½-inch rounds

2 zucchini, cut into ½-inch rounds

2 teaspoons vegan bouillon powder

2½ cups boiling water

scant ½ cup white wine

1⅓ cups frozen peas

12 cherry tomatoes

3 tablespoons finely chopped fresh mint leaves

3 tablespoons finely chopped fresh parsley

sea salt and ground black pepper

**1.** Preheat the oven to 350°F (180°C).

**2.** Place the pearl barley in the base of a high-sided oven tray. Add the fennel, potatoes, leeks, and zucchini to the barley.

**3.** Dissolve the bouillon in the boiling water and add the wine. Pour the liquid over the barley and vegetables and cover the tray with foil.

**4.** Bake for 30 minutes, then remove the foil, stir in the frozen peas, and distribute the cherry tomatoes over the top. Return to the oven for 20 minutes, uncovered.

**5.** To serve, stir in the finely chopped herbs and season.

# VEGAN MUSHROOM AND PUY LENTIL STROGANOFF

SERVES 2 | **Prep time:** 15 minutes | **Cook time:** 40 minutes
**Nutrition per serving:** 503 cal | 22.3g protein | 73.1g carbs | 61.1g fat | 11.2g fiber

*Adding nuts to a dish, particularly cashews, is a great way to create a creamy sauce without the use of dairy. The nuts don't just add flavor and texture but also promote a healthy cholesterol balance and are high in zinc to benefit the immune system.*

½ onion, finely diced

1 garlic clove, finely diced

1 carrot, finely diced

1½ celery sticks, finely diced

½ tablespoon olive oil

2 cups mushroom or vegetable stock

3 tablespoons raw cashew nuts

1 tablespoon chopped fresh tarragon

sea salt and ground black pepper

12½ ounces mushrooms (you can use any you like), chopped into bite-sized pieces

1 14-ounce can Puy lentils, drained and rinsed

⅔ cup cooked brown rice per serving

**1.** In a large pan, with a lid, cook the vegetables in ¼ tablespoon olive oil over medium heat for 5 minutes.

**2.** Add the stock and simmer for 10 minutes until the vegetables are soft. Pour the mixture into a blender with the cashew nuts and tarragon and blend until smooth and creamy. Season.

**3.** Return the pan to the heat, add the remaining ¼ tablespoon olive oil with the mushrooms, and stir regularly for 5 minutes until the mushrooms are cooked through. Add the lentils and the blended sauce and gently heat for another few minutes. Serve with the cooked brown rice or with a serving of green beans.

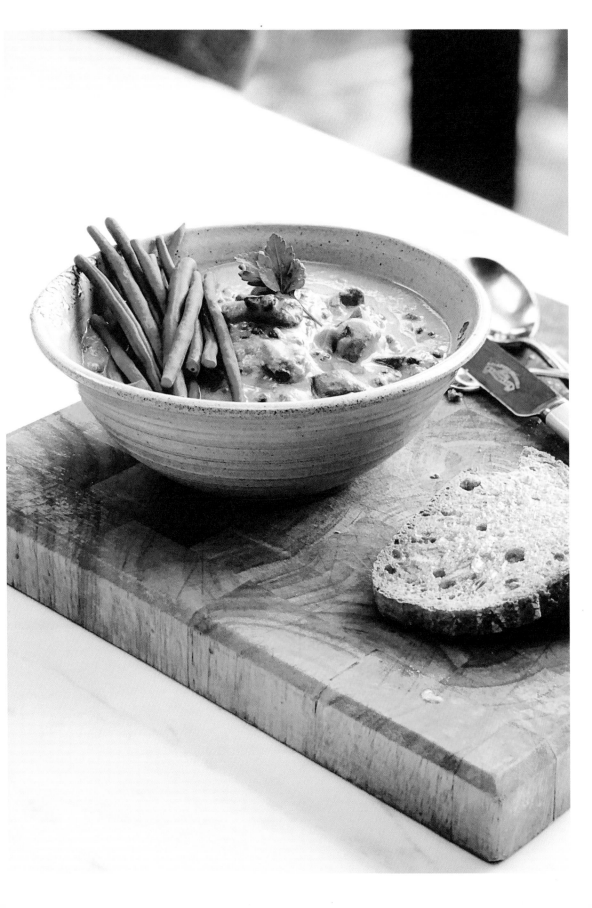

# VEGAN CAULIFLOWER "CHEESE" WITH SMOKY MUSHROOMS

SERVES 2 | **Prep time:** 20 minutes | **Cook time:** 20 minutes
**Nutrition per serving:** 341 cal | 17.4g protein | 34.8g carbs | 17.1g fat | 10.2g fiber

*The "cheese" sauce is another bit of plant-based magic, converting this classic comfort food into a dairy-free zone while drastically cutting the calories. It's important to use starchy, not waxy, potatoes; try Yukon Gold or Idaho.*

½ head of cauliflower, cut into florets

1 medium starchy potato (skin on), roughly chopped

1 carrot, roughly chopped

¼ cup nutritional yeast

1 tablespoon miso paste

⅓ cup raw cashew nuts

3 teaspoons Dijon mustard

¼ teaspoon garlic powder

¼ teaspoon onion powder

¼ teaspoon turmeric powder

ground black pepper, to taste

½ tablespoon olive oil

2 portobello mushrooms, sliced

½ teaspoon smoked paprika

**1.** Place the cauliflower florets in the top of a steamer pan. Place the potato and carrots in salted water in the bottom of the steamer pan. Bring to a boil and cook the vegetables for 10 minutes.

**2.** Place the cauliflower in an ovenproof dish. Transfer the potato and carrots to a blender with ¼ cup of the cooking water and the yeast, miso paste, cashews, mustard, garlic and onion powders, turmeric, and pepper. Blend the sauce for 30 seconds.

**3.** Preheat the broiler to high. Pour the sauce over the cauliflower and place under the broiler for 3–5 minutes.

**4.** Heat the olive oil in a pan and cook the mushrooms for 5 minutes, adding the smoked paprika 1 minute before they're fully cooked.

**5.** Top the broiled cauliflower "cheese" with the smoky mushrooms and serve.

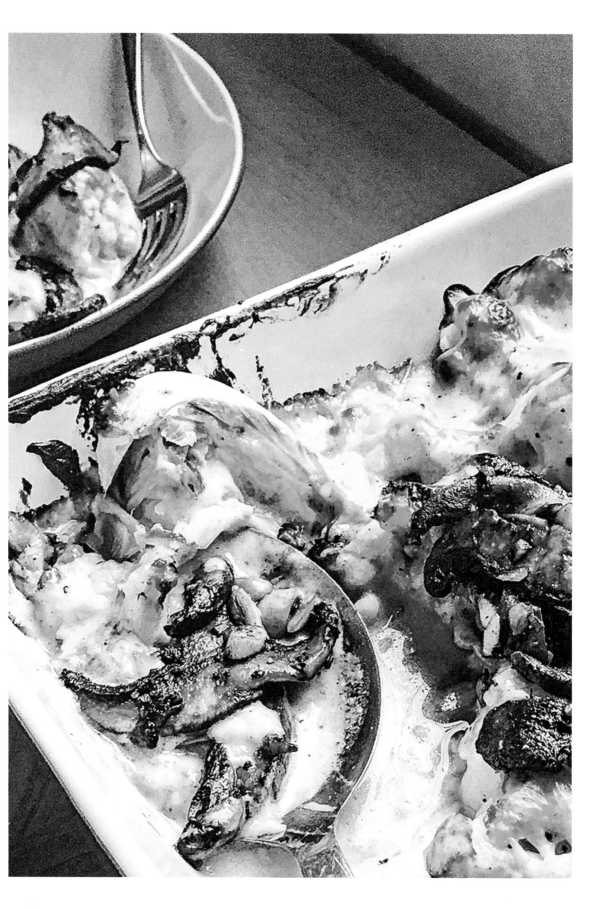

# PINEAPPLE, PEANUT, AND VEGETABLE CURRY

SERVES 2 | **Prep time:** 20 minutes | **Cook time:** 30 minutes
**Nutrition per serving:** 589 cal | 15.4g protein | 58.8g carbs | 32.9g fat | 6.6g fiber

½ onion, roughly chopped

1 garlic clove

thumb-sized piece fresh ginger, roughly chopped

1 fresh red chile

2 teaspoons garam masala

½ tablespoon coconut oil

pinch of salt

scant ⅔ cup chopped tomatoes

scant ⅔ cup coconut milk (from a can)

1 teaspoon vegan bouillon powder

1 tablespoon peanut butter

scant ½ cup water

2 ounces pineapple (fresh, frozen, or canned), chopped

1 head of bok choy, chopped

1½ ounces thin asparagus, chopped

⅓ cup unsalted peanuts

¾ cup cooked brown rice per serving

**1.** Place the onion, garlic, and ginger in a blender with the chile, garam masala, coconut oil, salt, and 2 tablespoons of water. Blend for around 20 seconds or until there are no lumps. Pour into a medium-sized pan over medium-high heat and cook for 5 minutes, stirring regularly.

**2.** Add the tomatoes, coconut milk, bouillon powder, and peanut butter to the blender and blend for 20 seconds until smooth. Pour over the onion and spice mix in the pan. Add the water to the blender, give it a quick pulse to collect the residue of the tomato-coconut mix, then add to the pan. Stir and bring to a boil, then reduce the heat and simmer for 20 minutes.

**3.** Add the pineapple, bok choy, asparagus, and peanuts to the cooked sauce and cook for a further 2–3 minutes to heat through, then serve with the cooked brown rice.

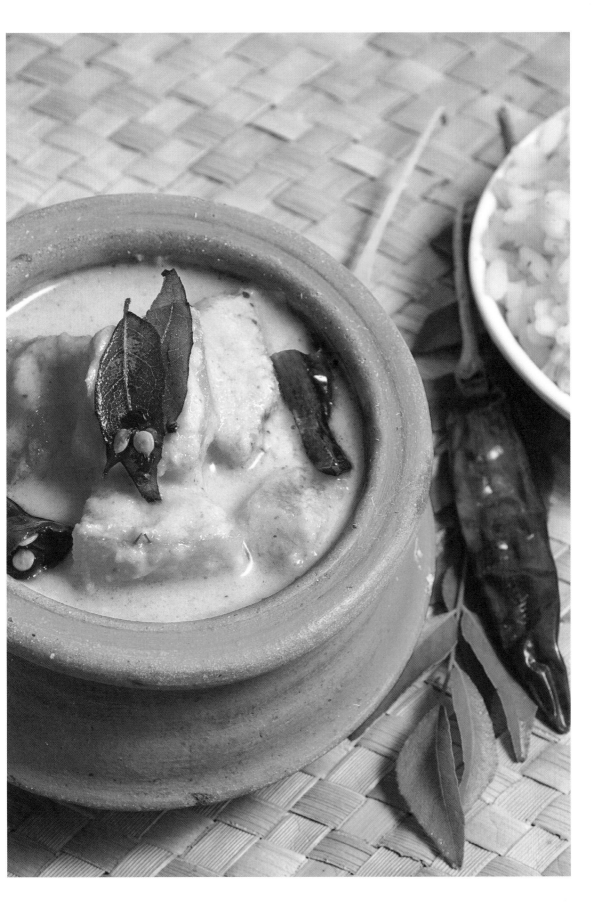

# PORCINI MUSHROOM AND THYME SPELTOTTO

SERVES 2 | **Prep time:** 10 minutes, plus 30 minutes' soaking time | **Cook time:** 50 minutes
**Nutrition per serving:** 343 cal | 14.2g protein | 47.8g carbs | 4.2g fat | 6.7g fiber

*Mushrooms are secret nutritional weapons that boost your immune system and feed your gut flora with prebiotics. Different types are beneficial in everything from energy production to mental health. This one-pot dish is packed full of mushrooms, and uses whole grain spelt instead of risotto rice.*

1½ ounces dried porcini
  mushrooms

1¾ cups boiling water

1 tablespoon olive oil

1 onion, finely chopped

3 garlic cloves

10 ounces portobello
  mushrooms, roughly chopped

1 cup spelt

½ cup white wine

2¾ cups water

2 mushroom stock cubes

6 sprigs of thyme

sea salt and ground black
  pepper

**1.** Place the dried mushrooms in a bowl and pour over the boiling water. Set aside to soak for 30 minutes.

**2.** In a large saucepan, heat the oil and cook the onion, garlic, and fresh mushrooms for 5–10 minutes until softened. Add the soaked mushrooms and all the other ingredients except the salt and pepper. Bring to a boil, then reduce the heat and simmer for around 40 minutes, stirring occasionally and adding more water if it starts to get too dry. It should be moist and have a creamy texture. Cook until the spelt is plump and well cooked.

**3.** Once cooked, discard the thyme twigs, season, and serve.

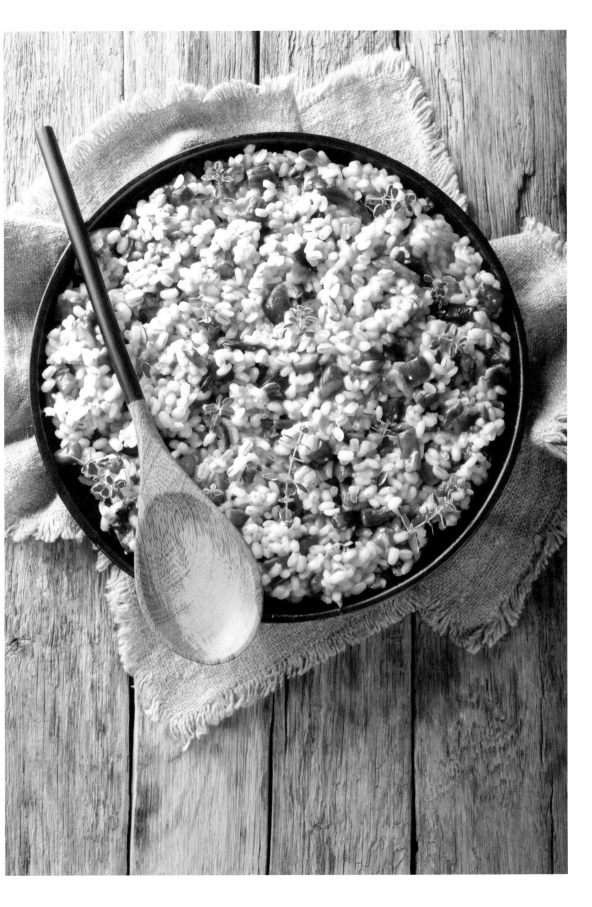

# INDEX

# RECIPE FINDER